Nutritional Abnormalities in Infectious Diseases: Effects on Tuberculosis and AIDS

Nutrional Immunology series:

Vitamin A and the Immune Function: A Symposium, edited by Chris Kjolhede and William
    R. Beisel

Nutritional Abnormalities in Infectious Diseases: Effects on Tuberculosis and AIDS

Christopher E. Taylor, ScD
Editor

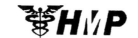

The Haworth Medical Press
An Imprint of
The Haworth Press, Inc.
New York

Published by

The Haworth Medical Press, 10 Alice Street, Binghamton, NY 13904-1580

The Haworth Medical Press is an imprint of the Haworth Press, Inc., 10 Alice Street, Binghamton, NY 13904-1580 USA.

Nutritional Abnormalities in Infectious Diseases: Effects on Tuberculosis and AIDS has also been published as *Journal of Nutritional Immunology,* Volume 5, Number 1 1997.

The development, preparation, and publication of this work has been undertaken with great care. However, the publisher, employees, editors, and agents of The Haworth Press and all imprints of The Haworth Press, Inc., including The Haworth Medical Press and Pharmaceutical Products Press, are not responsible for any errors contained herein or for consequences that may ensue from use of materials or information contained in this work. Opinions expressed by the author(s) are not necessarily those of The Haworth Press, Inc.

Library of Congress Cataloging-in-Publication Data

Nutritional abnormalities in infectious diseases: effects on tuberculosis and AIDS / Christopher E. Taylor, editor.

   p. cm.

  Published also as Journal of nutritional immunology; v. 5, no. 1.

  Includes bibliographical references and index.

  ISBN 0-7890-0019-9

  1. AIDS (Disease)–Nutritional aspects. 2. Tuberculosis–Nutritional aspects. 3. Malnutrition–Complications. 4. Immunity–Nutritional aspects. I. Taylor, Christopher E.

  [DNLM: 1. Nutrition Disorders–complications. 2. Tuberculosis–complications. 3. Acquired Immunodeficiency Syndrome–complications. 4. Nutrition. W1 JO798HS v. 5 no. 1 1997 / WD 100 N97557 1997]

RC607.A26N89 1997

616.97′92–dc21

DNLM/DLC

for Library of Congress

96-51894

CIP

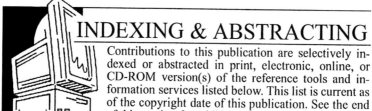

INDEXING & ABSTRACTING

Contributions to this publication are selectively indexed or abstracted in print, electronic, online, or CD-ROM version(s) of the reference tools and information services listed below. This list is current as of the copyright date of this publication. See the end of this section for additional notes.

- *AGRICOLA Database,* National Agricultural Library, 10301 Baltimore Boulevard, Room 002, Beltsville, MD 20705

- *Biology Digest,* Plexus Publishing Company, 143 Old Marlton Pike, Medford, NJ 08055

- *Biosciences Information Service of Biological Abstracts (BIOSIS),* Biosciences Information Service, 2100 Arch Street, Philadelphia, PA 19103-1399

- *Biostatistica,* Executive Sciences Institute, 1005 Mississippi Avenue, Davenport, IA 52803

- *Cambridge Scientific Abstracts, Health & Safety Science Abstracts*, Enviromental Routenet (accessed via INTERNET), 7200 Wisconsin Avenue #601, Bethesda, MD 20814

- *Chemical Abstracts,* Chemical Abstracts Service Library, 2540 Olgentangy Road, P.O. Box 3012, Columbus, OH 43210

- *Child Development Abstracts & Bibliography,* University of Kansas, 2 Bailey Hall, Lawrence, KS 66045

- *CNPIEC Reference Guide: Chinese National Directory of Foreign Periodicals,* P.O. Box 88, Beijing, People's Republic of China

- *Combined Health Information Database (CHID)*, National Institutes of Health, 3 Information Way, Bethesda, MD 20892-3580

- *CPcurrents,* ITServices, 3301 Alta Arden #3, Sacramento, CA 95825

- *Current Awareness in Biological Sciences (C.A.B.S),* 3 Saxby Street, Christopher Mews, Leicester LE2 0AZ, UK

- *Current Contents* . . . . . see Institute for Scientific Information

(continued)

- *Excerpta Medica/Secondary Publishing Division,* Elsevier Science Inc., Secondary Publishing Division, 655 Avenue of the Americas, New York, NY 10010

- *Food Science and Technology Abstracts (FSTA),* scanned, abstracted and indexed by the International Food Information Service (IFIS) for inclusion in Food Science and Technology Abstracts (FSTA), International Food Information Service, Land End House, Shinfield, Reading RG2 9BB, England

- *Foods Adlibra,* Foods Adlibra Publications, 9000 Plymouth Avenue North, Minneapolis, MN 55427

- *Greenfiles,* 138 Oak Tree Lane, Nottinghamshire NG18 3HR, UK

- *Index to Periodical Articles Related to Law,* University of Texas, 727 East 26th Street, Austin, TX 78705

- *Institute for Scientific Information,* 3501 Market Street, Philadelphia, Pennsylvania 19104. Coverage in:
  a) Social Science Citation Index [SSCI]: print, online, CD-ROM
  b) Research Alerts [current awareness service]
  c) Social SciSearch [magnetic tape]
  d) Current Contents/Social & Behavioral Sciences [weekly current awaremess service]

- *INTERNET ACCESS (& additional networks) Bulletin Board for Libraries ("BUBL"), coverage of information resources on INTERNET, JANET, and other networks.*
  - JANET X.29: UK.AC.BATH.BUBL or 00006012101300
  - TELNET: BUBL.BATH.AC.UK or 138.38.32.45 login 'bubl'
  - Gopher: BUBL.BATH.AC.UK (138.32.32.45). Port 7070
  - World Wide Web: http: / / www.bubl.bath.ac.uk./BUBL/ home.html
  - NISSWAIS: telnetniss.ac.uk (for the NISS gateway)
  The Andersonian Library, Curran Building, 101 St. James Road, Glasgow G4 ONS, Scotland

- *Natural Products Alert (NAPRALERT),* University of Illinois at Chicago, 833 South Wood Street, Chicago, IL 60612

- *Nutrition Abstracts & Reviews Series (NARS/CAB ABSTRACTS),* B–Livestock Feeds & Feeding; Nutrition Abstracts & Reviews Series A–Human & Experimental, c/o CAB International/CAB ACCESS . . . available in print, diskettes updated weekly, and on INTERNET. Providing full bibliographic listings, author affiliation, augmented keyword searching. CAB International, P.O. Box 100, Wallingford Oxon OX10 8DE, UK

(continued)

- *Nutrition Research Newsletter "Abstracts Section,"* Lyda Associates, Inc., P.O. Box 700, Palisades, NY 10964

- *Referativnyi Zhurnal (Abstracts Journal of the Institute of Scientific Information of the Republic of Russia),* The Institute of Scientific Information, Baltijskaja ul., 14, Moscow A-219, Republic of Russia

- *Wildlife Review/Fisheries Review,* US Fish and Wildlife Service, 1201 Oak Ridge Drive, Suite 200, Fort Collins, CO 80525-5589

SPECIAL BIBLIOGRAPHIC NOTES

*related to special journal issues (separates)
and indexing/abstracting*

❏ indexing/abstracting services in this list will also cover material in any "separate" that is co-published simultaneously with Haworth's special thematic journal issue or DocuSerial. Indexing/abstracting usually covers material at the article/chapter level.

❏ monographic co-editions are intended for either non-subscribers or libraries which intend to purchase a second copy for their circulating collections.

❏ monographic co-editions are reported to all jobbers/wholesalers/approval plans. The source journal is listed as the "series" to assist the prevention of duplicate purchasing in the same manner utilized for books-in-series.

❏ to facilitate user/access services all indexing/abstracting services are encouraged to utilize the co-indexing entry note indicated at the bottom of the first page of each article/chapter/contribution.

❏ this is intended to assist a library user of any reference tool (whether print, electronic, online, or CD-ROM) to locate the monographic version if the library has purchased this version but not a subscription to the source journal.

❏ individual articles/chapters in any Haworth publication are also available through the Haworth Document Delivery Services (HDDS).

Nutritional Abnormalities in Infectious Diseases: Effects on Tuberculosis and AIDS

CONTENTS

∞ ALL HAWORTH MEDICAL PRESS BOOKS
AND JOURNALS ARE PRINTED
ON CERTIFIED ACID-FREE PAPER

ABOUT THE EDITOR

Christopher E. Taylor, ScD, is Program Officer in the Respiratory Diseases Branch, Division of Microbiology and Infectious Diseases, and former Senior Staff Fellow in the Laboratory of Immunogenetics, at the National Institute of Allergy and Infectious Diseases. Prior to that he was Assistant Professor in the Department of Microbiology and Immunology at the Medical College of Pennsylvania. Dr. Taylor has served as Chair of the Immunology Division and of the Divisional Symposium of the American Society for Microbiology and is active in other professional societies, including the American Association of Immunology and the American Association for Advancement of Science. His research interests include antibody and cytokine responses to bacterial pathogens.

Introduction

Christopher E. Taylor, ScD

Tuberculosis (TB) is responsible for significant mortality and morbidity worldwide and it has been estimated that the disease will claim more than 30 million lives in the coming decade. For a while it was presumed that chemotherapy was sufficient to control the disease. However, because of the recent emergence of multidrug resistant strains and the lack of patient adherence to therapy it is now clear, especially in the light of the growing numbers of TB cases, that alternative approaches must be taken. Indeed, the eventual outcome of the host-mycobacterial interaction depends on several complex factors including genetic, environmental, and nutritional conditions. It was the intent of this round table to focus specifically on the nutritional factors in an effort to:

1. Identify the most crucial nutritional determinants involved in the control of TB;
2. Outline the nutrient sensitive host defense mechanisms involved, including the role of cytokines;
3. Define the effects of malabsorption and drug-drug interactions; and
4. Demonstrate the effects of co-infection with HIV on the incidence of TB.

Christopher E. Taylor, Program Officer, Respiratory Diseases Branch, Division of Microbiology and Infectious Diseases, National Institute of Allergy and Infectious Diseases, Rockville, MD.

Address correspondence to: Christopher E. Taylor, ScD, Respiratory Diseases Branch, Division of Microbiology and Infectious Diseases, NIAID, 6003 Executive Boulevard, Solar Building, Room 3B01, Bethesda, MD 20892-7630.

[Haworth co-indexing entry note]: "Introduction." Christopher E. Taylor. Co-published simultaneously in *Journal of Nutritional Immunology* (The Haworth Medical Press, an imprint of The Haworth Press, Inc.) Vol. 5, No. 1, 1997, p. 1; and: *Nutritional Abnormalities in Infectious Diseases: Effects on Tuberculosis and AIDS* (ed: Christopher E. Taylor) The Haworth Medical Press, an imprint of The Haworth Press, Inc., 1997, p. 1. Single or multiple copies of this article are available for a fee from The Haworth Document Delivery Service [1-800-342-9678, 9:00 a.m. - 5:00 p.m. (EST). E-mail address: getinfo@haworth.com].

Nutritional Determinants of Resistance to Tuberculosis

David N. McMurray, PhD

The relationship between malnutrition and tuberculosis is probably as ancient as the disease itself. The global tuberculosis problem, which never has been addressed adequately, has always included chronic undernutrition as an inescapable concomitant.[1] The long-standing importance of reactivation disease in the elderly, coupled in the past 10 years with a dramatic re-emergence of primary tuberculosis in this country, has focused attention on the interaction between nutritional status and tuberculosis resistance.[2] It is not mere coincidence that many of the high risk groups for tuberculosis in the U.S., e.g., the elderly, the homeless, drug abusers, alcoholics, the institutionalized, and HIV-infected individuals, are also high risk groups for nutritional deficiencies.[3]

The results of early research on the effect of dietary deficiencies and resistance to infection with mycobacteria were summarized in a review published in 1968.[4] Table 1 demonstrates that the vast majority of those studies, involving humans and various experimental animal species and a variety of essential nutrients, documented a synergistic (i.e., detrimental) interaction in which the nutrient-de-

David N. McMurray, Department of Medical Microbiology and Immunology, Texas A&M University, College Station, TX.

Address correspondence to David N. McMurray, PhD, Texas A&M University, 407 Reynolds Building, College Station, TX 77845-1114.

[Haworth co-indexing entry note]: "Nutritional Determinants of Resistance to Tuberculosis." McMurray, David N. Co-published simultaneously in *Journal of Nutritional Immunology* (The Haworth Medical Press, an imprint of The Haworth Press, Inc.) Vol. 5, No. 1, 1997, pp. 3-10; and: *Nutritional Abnormalities in Infectious Diseases: Effects on Tuberculosis and AIDS* (ed: Christopher E. Taylor) The Haworth Medical Press, an imprint of The Haworth Press, Inc., 1997, pp. 3-10. Single or multiple copies of this article are available for a fee from The Haworth Document Delivery Service [1-800-342-9678, 9:00 a.m. - 5:00 p.m. (EST). E-mail address: getinfo@haworth.com].

TABLE 1. Impact of Nutritional Deficiencies on Tuberculosis (1923-1961)*

Dietary Deficiency	Species	Total Number of Studies	Type of Interaction		
			Synergistic	Antagonistic	None
Multiple	mouse, guinea pig, human	9	8	0	1
Protein	mouse, rat, guinea pig, human, hamster	18	1	3	4
Vitamin C	guinea pig, human	8	8	0	0
Vitamin A	mouse, rat, human, chicken	4	4	0	0
Vitamin D	mouse	1	0	0	1

*Based upon N. S. Scrimshaw et al.[4]

prived individuals expressed reduced resistance to infection with *Mycobacterium tuberculosis*. More recently, a number of other nutrients have been implicated in the immune response to tubercle bacilli, either *in vivo* or *in vitro*. These include protein,[5] iron,[6] vitamin D,[7] retinol,[8] vitamin B_{12},[9] and others.

In the last 20 years, a large and impressive body of literature has been generated which demonstrates that experimental deficiencies of nearly every essential nutrient can produce impairment of some aspect of immunologic function.[10,11] The relevance of many of these observations for infectious disease resistance is difficult to assess, however, because relatively few studies included actual infection of the nutrient-deprived animals. In fact, it is clear that resistance to some obligate intracellular microbes, which are intimately dependent upon host cell metabolic processes, may actually be increased in malnutrition. Therefore, it may be misleading to extrapolate from detrimental effects of malnutrition on immune response to alteration in disease resistance.

A priori, one can identify several aspects of the pathogenesis of tuberculosis which might be sensitive to nutritional insult. These include the physiological state of the alveoli and their resident macrophages, the delivery (or denial) of essential nutrients and substrates to intracellular mycobacteria, the activation, expansion, cytokine production and trafficking of protective CD4$^+$ and CD8$^+$ T lymphocytes, the ability of macrophages to become activated to produce microbicidal reactive oxygen and nitrogen intermediates, the formation of mature granulomas, and the delicately balanced immunoregulatory networks involving T cell subsets producing specific cytokine profiles. Although many of these host immune functions have been shown to be sensitive to nutrient deprivation in infected animals, few have been examined in the context of infection with *M. tuberculosis* or other human pathogens.

One approach to the identification of nutritional determinants of resistance to tuberculosis has been to utilize a guinea pig model of low-dose pulmonary infection with virulent *M. tuberculosis*.[12] This model system mimics many of the important features of primary tuberculosis in humans, such as the development of a few primary lung granulomas, a bacillemic phase leading to reseeding of the lung by the hematogenous route, the expression of strong T cell-mediated immunity *in vivo* and *in vitro*, and the ability of guinea pigs to acquire solid resistance following vaccination.[13,14] This model system has been used over the past 10 years to examine the impact of dietary deficiencies of protein, zinc, and vitamin D on both BCG vaccine-induced and innate resistance to virulent tubercle bacilli.

Of all of the nutrients examined with respect to their impact on immunity, zinc deficiency has demonstrated a dramatic and consistent detrimental effect on thymus-dependent immune functions in both humans and animals.[15] Guinea pigs fed for several weeks on a markedly zinc-deficient diet developed the classic signs of zinc deficiency, including reduced food intake and weight loss, thymic atrophy and serum Zn levels less than half those in zinc-replete controls.[16] Upon infection with *M. tuberculosis*, zinc-deficient guinea pigs failed to develop delayed hypersensitivity reactions following intradermal injection of PPD. Zinc-deprived, tuberculous animals had significant reductions in the number of circulating T cells and impaired PPD-induced proliferation *in vitro*.[17] Production of macrophage migration inhibition factor (MIF) was unaffected by zinc status.[18] In spite of the T cell defects suggestive of loss of protective functions, infection of zinc-deficient BCG-vaccinated and nonvaccinated guinea pigs with virulent *M. tuberculosis* by the respiratory route resulted in no change in resistance as expressed in terms of mycobacterial loads in the lung and spleen. Thus, a level of zinc deficiency sufficient to produce altered peripheral T cell function did not influence the ability of the animals to control mycobacterial replication.

The activated form of vitamin D_3, $1,25(OH)_2$ D_3 or calcitriol, is produced by activated macrophages and may act synergistically with γIFN to retard intracellular replication of mycobacteria.[7,19] Different levels of vitamin D deficiency were produced by feeding guinea pigs diets containing 50%, 25% or 0% of the recommended dietary level (1180 IU/kg) for several weeks. Confirmation of the effect of the deficient diets on vitamin D metabolism *in vivo* was obtained by measuring circulating levels of the principal vitamin D metabolite, $25(OH)D_3$. The results of these studies[17,20] demonstrate that chronic dietary vitamin D deficiency did exert a detrimental effect on antigen (PPD)-specific T cell responses in tuberculous guinea pigs. Both dermal tuberculin reactions and PPD-induced lymphoproliferation *in vitro* were significantly less intense in vitamin D-deprived animals. However, vitamin D-deprived guinea pigs responded to pulmonary infection with virulent *M. tuberculosis* by allowing exactly the same degree of bacterial accumulation in the lung and spleen as that seen in well-nourished counterparts. Likewise, prior vaccination with BCG protected both groups of guinea pigs identically.[20] These results reveal that a degree of dietary vitamin D deficiency sufficient to produce significant alterations in PPD-specific T cell functions *in vivo* and *in vitro* did not alter the level of innate or vaccine-induced resistance to virulent *M. tuberculosis* in this model.

A state of chronic, moderate protein deficiency was produced by feeding guinea pigs a diet containing about one-third of their protein requirement for several weeks. Protein deficiency in young, growing animals was characterized by significantly reduced growth velocity, decreased serum albumin levels, atrophy of lymphoid organs, loss of subcutaneous fat and muscle mass, and edema.[5] Upon infection with virulent mycobacteria, protein-deprived guinea pigs exhibited dramatic loss of T cell functions *in vivo* and *in vitro*, reductions in the proportion of circulating $CD2^+$ T cells, redistribution of $CD4^+$ and $CD8^+$ T cell subsets, and decreased IL-2 production and response to exogenous recombinant IL-2 *in vitro*.[21-23] Interestingly, activity of another cytokine (MIF) was also adversely affected in protein-deprived guinea pigs.[18] More importantly, protein malnourished guinea pigs failed to respond to BCG vaccination as vigorously as well-nourished control animals. BCG vaccine efficacy, as measured by reductions in the bacterial loads in the lung and spleen 3-5 weeks post-challenge, was impaired partially or completely (Figure 1). Innate resistance to pulmonary challenge did not seem to be affected as dramatically. Recent experiments involving adoptive transfer of immune cells between normal and malnourished donor and recipient inbred guinea pigs point to defects in T cell trafficking, clonal expansion *in vivo,* and subset balance as possible explanations for the loss of vaccine-induced resistance to tuberculosis in protein deficiency.[23]

Taken together, these results demonstrate that dietary deficiencies of zinc, vitamin D, and protein are associated with remarkably similar defects in antigen-specific T cell responses *in vivo* and in

FIGURE 1. Degree of protection (reduction in mean $\log_{10}$ number of viable *M. tuberculosis*) afforded by prior BCG vaccination to control and protein-deficient guinea pigs 4 wk after pulmonary challenge. Mean ± SEM of 3-4 animals per diet treatment; asterisk denotes significant diet effect ($P < 0.05$).

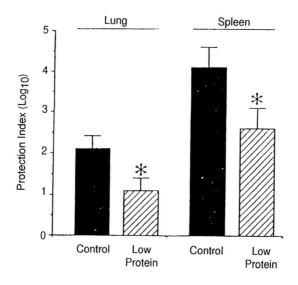

vitro, in guinea pigs infected with virulent *M. tuberculosis*. While it might have been tempting to speculate about the significance of these T cell defects for disease resistance, actual challenge studies under highly relevant conditions revealed that only one of the dietary deficiencies (i.e., protein) was actually accompanied by loss of tuberculosis resistance following BCG vaccination. This somewhat unexpected outcome illustrates the importance of including microbial infection in dietary studies to confirm the biological significance of the immunological deficits observed.

The second important conclusion from these studies is that diet can be a fundamental determinant of the host-parasite interaction in tuberculosis. These results, obtained in a model which mimics closely the events in human disease, support the hypothesis that chronic protein deprivation likely contributed to the disappointing outcome often observed in BCG field trials in developing countries.[24] Furthermore, these results suggest that protein malnutrition may significantly affect resistance to tuberculosis in the elderly, cachectic HIV+ individuals, alcoholics, the homeless, and other high risk groups in this country who are marginalized socially and economically. An extensive research effort will be required to elucidate the mechanisms by which protein and other crucial nutrients impair disease resistance, and to test novel nutritional and immunomodulatory approaches to augmenting the resistance of malnourished patients.

REFERENCES

1. Sudre, P., ten Dam, G., and Kochi, A. (1992). Tuberculosis: A global overview of the situation today. Bull. Wrld. Hlth. Org., 70:149-159.

2. Bloom, B.R. and Murray, C.J.L. (1992) Tuberculosis: Commentary on a reemergent killer. Science 757:1055-1064.

3. Collins, F. M. (1993). Tuberculosis: The return of an old enemy. Crit. Rev. Microbiol. 19:1-16.

4. Scrimshaw, N.S., Taylor, C.E., and Gordon, J.E. (1968). Interactions of nutrition and infection. WHO Monograph Series No. 57, World Health Organization, Geneva, Switzerland, pp. 60-329.

5. McMurray, D.N. and Yetley, E.A. (1983). Response to *Mycobacterium bovis* BCG vaccination in protein- and zinc-deficient guinea pigs. Infect. Immun. 39:755-761.

6. Douvas, G.S., May, M.H., and Crowle, A.J. (1993). Transferrin, iron and serum lipids enhance or inhibit *Mycobacterium avium* replication in human macrophages. J. Infect. Dis. 167:857-864.

7. Rook, G.A.W., Steele, J., Fraher, L., Barker, S., Karmali, R., O'Riordan, J., and Stanford, J. (1986). Vitamin D3, gamma interferon, and control of proliferation of *Mycobacterium tuberculosis* by human monocytes. Immunol. 57:159-163.

8. Crowle, A.H. and Ross, E.J. (1989). Inhibition by retinoic acid of multiplication of virulent tubercle bacilli in cultured human macrophages. Infect. Immun., 57:840-844.

9. Chanarin, I. and Stephenson, E. (1988). Vegetarian diet and cobalamin deficiency: their association with tuberculosis. J. Clin. Pathol. 41:759-762.

10. Chandra, R.K. (Ed.). (1988). *Nutrition and Immunology*. Alan R. Liss, New York, N.Y.

11. Cunningham-Rundes, S. (Ed.). (1993). *Nutrient Modulation of the Immune Response*, Marcel Dekker, New York, NY.

12. Smith, D.W. and Harding, G.E. (1977). Animal model of human disease. Pulmonary tuberculosis. Am. J. Pathol. 84:273-276.

13. Smith, D.W. and Wiegeshaus, E.H. (1989). What animal models can teach us about the pathogenesis of tuberculosis in humans. Rev. Infect. Dis. 11:S385-S393.

14. Wiegeshaus, E.H., Balasubramanian, V., and Smith, D.W. (1989). Immunity to tuberculosis from the perspective of pathogenesis. Infect. Immun. 57: 3671-3676.

15. Vruwink, K.G., Keen, C.L., Gershwin, M.E., Mareschi, J.P., and Hurley, L.S. (1993). The effect of experimental zinc deficiency on development of the immune system. In: Cunningham-Rundles, S. (ed.), *Nutrient modulation of the immune response*, Marcel Dekker, New York, NY, pp. 263-279.

16. McMurray, D.N., Carlomagno, M.A., and Cumberland, P.A. (1983). Respiratory infection with attenuated *Mycobacterium tuberculosis* H37Ra in malnourished guinea pigs. Infect. Immun., 39:793-799.

17. McMurray, D.N., Bartow, R.A., Mintzer, C.L. and Hernandez-Frontera, E. (1990). Micronutrient status and immune function in tuberculosis. Ann. N.Y. Acad. Sc. 587:59-69.

18. Carlomagno, M.A., Mintzer, C.L., Tetzlaff, C.L., and McMurray, D.N. (1985). Differential effect of protein and zinc deficiencies on delayed hypersensitivity and lymphokine activity in BCG-vaccinated guinea pigs. Nutr. Res. 5:959-968.

19. Rook, G.A.W. (1988). The role of vitamin D in tuberculosis. Am. Rev. Resp. Dis. 138:768-770.

20. Hernandez-Frontera, E. and McMurray, D.N. (1993). Dietary vitamin D affects cell-mediated hypersensitivity but not resistance to experimental pulmonary tuberculosis in guinea pigs. Infect. Immun. 61:2116-2121.

21. McMurray, D.N., Bartow, R.A., and Mintzer, C. (1990). Malnutrition-induced impairment of resistance against experimental pulmonary tuberculosis. In: Seminara, D., Pawlowski, A. and Watson, R. (Eds.); *Alcohol, immunomodulation and AIDS*, Alan R. Liss Inc., New York, NY, pp. 403-412.

22. McMurray, D.N. and Bartow, R.A. (1992). Immunosuppression and alteration of resistance to pulmonary tuberculosis in guinea pigs by protein undernutrition. J. Nutr. 122:738-743.

23. McMurray, D.N., Mainali, E.S., and Phalen, S. (1993). Malnutrition, immunoregulatory defects and the white plague. Adv. Biosci. 86:19-28.

24. Smith, D.W. (1985). Protective effect of BCG in experimental tuberculosis. Adv. Tuberc. Res. 22:1-97.

Effects of Protein Calorie Malnutrition on Mice Infected with BCG

J. Chan, MD
K. Tanaka, MD
C. Mannion, MD
D. Carroll, BSc
M. Tsang, BSc
Y. Xing, MD
C. Lowenstein, MD
Barry R. Bloom, PhD

Tuberculosis has been linked historically to poor nutritional status such as protein calorie malnutrition (PCM).[1] The wasting character of tuberculosis, denoted by terms like "phthisis" (Greek for "wasting away") and "consumption," has been well documented.[2] As a major cause of morbidity and mortality in developing countries where PCM is also highly prevalent,[3,4] tuberculosis is one of the model diseases whose pathogenesis has been examined in the

J. Chan is affiliated with the Department of Medicine; K. Tanaka, C. Mannion, and D. Carroll are affiliated with the Department of Pathology; M. Tsang and Y. Xing are affiliated with the Department of Medicine, Montefiore Medical Center, Albert Einstein College of Medicine, Bronx, NY. C. Lowenstein is affiliated with the Department of Medicine, Johns Hopkins University School of Medicine, Baltimore, MD. Barry R. Bloom is affiliated with the Howard Hughes Medical Institute, Albert Einstein College of Medicine, Bronx, NY.

Address correspondence to: J. Chan, MD, Department of Medicine, Centennial Floor, Montefiore Medical Center, 111 E. 210th Street, Bronx, NY 10467.

[Haworth co-indexing entry note]: "Effects of Protein Calorie Malnutrition on Mice Infected with BCG." Chan, J. et al. Co-published simultaneously in *Journal of Nutritional Immunology* (The Haworth Medical Press, an imprint of The Haworth Press, Inc.) Vol. 5, No. 1, 1997, pp. 11-19; and: *Nutritional Abnormalities in Infectious Diseases: Effects on Tuberculosis and AIDS* (ed: Christopher E. Taylor) The Haworth Medical Press, an imprint of The Haworth Press, Inc., 1997, pp. 11-19. Single or multiple copies of this article are available for a fee from The Haworth Document Delivery Service [1-800-342-9678, 9:00 a.m. - 5:00 p.m. (EST). E-mail address: getinfo@haworth.com].

context of malnutrition in many laboratories using various animal experimental tuberculosis models. Despite such efforts, the mechanisms underlying the association between PCM and exacerbation of tuberculous infection are not clearly defined. Nonetheless, as evidence accumulates that PCM induces secondary immunodeficiency, particularly cellular immunity,[4,5] much effort has been focused on examining the mechanisms of how dysfunction of the cellular immune response secondary to dietary protein deficiency causes increased susceptibility to tuberculous infection.[5] The present study provides evidence that deficiencies exist in two cellular immune defense mechanisms in protein calorie malnourished mice during BCG infection: (i) the expression of nitric oxide synthase, the enzyme that mediates a major antimycobacterial effector mechanism of macrophages[6-8] and (ii) the formation of granuloma, an immuological response generally accepted as critical in defense against mycobacterial infection.

The Role of Reactive Nitrogen Intermediates (RNI) in Host Defense Against M. tuberculosis

The L-arginine-dependent cytotoxic pathway of cytokine-activated murine macrophages has recently been shown to kill *Mycobacterium* spp. effectively *in vitro*, including virulent strains of *M. tuberculosis*.[8] The cytostatic and cytocidal effects of this antimicrobial mechanism, inducible by interferon-gamma (IFN-γ) and tumor necrosis factor-alpha (TNF-α),[9] as well as bacterial products such as *E. coli* lipopolysaccharide (LPS)[10] and mycobacterial lipoarabinnomannan (LAM),[11] are mediated via nitric oxide and related reactive nitrogen intermediates (RNI). These toxic nitrogen oxides are generated by the inducible isoform of nitric oxide synthase (iNOS) of macrophages using the substrate L-arginine. Exploiting transgenic murine models that utilize animals with targeted disruption of the genes for IFN-γ receptor,[12] IFN-γ,[13-15] or IFN-γ regulatory factor-1,[16] we and others have provided experimental evidence that this antimicrobial pathway plays a critical role in host defense against mycobacterial infection *in vivo*. The significance of RNI in mycobacterial diseases *in vivo* is further reinforced by results from our laboratory demonstrating that inhibitors of NOS markedly exacerbate *M. tuberculosis* infection in mice.[17] In the latter study, two distinct NOS inhibitors, aminoguanidine and N[G]monomethyl-L-arginine were used in the same murine tuberculosis model, and both rendered similar deleterious effects on disease progression in mice infected with the virulent Erdman strain of *M. tuberculosis*, thus strongly implicating the nitric oxide generating pathway as a major defense mechanism against *M. tuberculosis in vivo*.

Effects of Protein Calorie Malnutrition on CD1 Mice Infected with BCG

One strategy to evaluate the significance of RNI generated via the L-arginine-dependent cytotoxic pathway in resistance against mycobacteria *in vivo* is to compare the relative virulence of the tubercle bacillus in animals that differ in their ability to produce toxic RNI. In an attempt to render animals deficient in RNI production, we chose initially to deplete L-arginine, the natural substrate for NOS, through diet manipulation. In the course of these experiments, it was observed that diet deficient solely in L-arginine had no apparent effect on BCG infection in relatively resistant CD1 mice. We reasoned that this observation was likely because endogenous production of L-arginine was sufficient to provide an adequate amount of this amino acid for macrophage iNOS to generate RNI in response to BCG infection.[18] In contrast, it was observed that BCG infection followed a fulminant course in mice fed a protein-deficient diet. Since it is known that RNI plays a significant role in host defense against mycobacteria, this murine PCM model was exploited to examine the relationship between dietary protein deficiency, exacerbation of mycobacterial infection, and expression of the L-arginine-dependent cytotoxic pathway.

In these experiments, eight-to-ten-week-old CD1 female mice were used. Protein calorie malnutrition was achieved using a 2% protein diet. This protein-deficient diet was made isocaloric as the control normal diet by carbohydrate supplementation. The 2% protein diet was chosen based on preliminary results indicating that this dietary protein content rendered CD1 mice more susceptible to BCG infection as assessed by tissue bacterial burden and morbidity. Control animals given the same diet without infection survived for up to 6 months without apparent distress. Mice were infected with 1×10^6 BCG (strain Pasteur) intravenously via the lateral tail vein, as previously described,[14] 10 to 14 days after initiation of the protein-deficient diet. At various time intervals post-infection, the expression of the L-arginine-dependent cytotoxic pathway in BCG-infected mice were examined directly by immunohistochemical staining using an affinity purified antibody specific for macrophage iNOS. Standardization experiments revealed that expression of macrophage iNOS in the tissues of BCG-infected mice was almost exclusively localized to the granulomatous lesions, suggesting that activation of the RNI-generating pathway during infection is a highly regulated process.

Immunohistochemical staining of the tissues from mice fed 2% and full protein diet demonstrated a striking difference in the expression of macrophage iNOS (Figure 1). While mice fed a normal protein diet expressed macrophage iNOS in the liver 3 to 5 days after infection, the ability of the protein malnourished animals to do so was markedly depressed. This remarkable difference continued for at least 10 days post-infection. By day 14 after the initiation of infection, the difference in iNOS expression in the liver between the two groups of mice appeared to have normalized. Similarly, a difference in iNOS expression between the protein calorie malnourished animals and those fed a normal diet was also observed in the lungs (Figure 2). This latter observation must, however, be interpreted with caution due to the paucity of pulmonary granulomas as a result of the relatively small number of bacilli ($\sim$1% of the inoculum) delivered to the lungs via the intravenous route.[19] Parallel examination of histologic sections indicate that granulomatous lesions of mice with PCM were poorly formed compared to that of animals fed a normal diet (Figure 2). This finding had been observed previously in another murine model of BCG infection.[20] In addition, the number of BCG in tissues of malnourished mice, as shown by Kinyoun's acid fast stain, far exceeded that found in well-nourished mice (Figure 3). Finally, increased mortality was observed in BCG-infected mice fed the protein deficient diet (data not shown). Preliminary data in our laboratory indicate that infection of protein calorie malnourished animals with virulent *M. tuberculosis* results in a highly fulminant and rapidly fatal disease.

Taken together, these results reveal defects in two cellular defense mechanisms that may account for the increased susceptibility to mycobacterial infection in mice with PCM. First, expression of

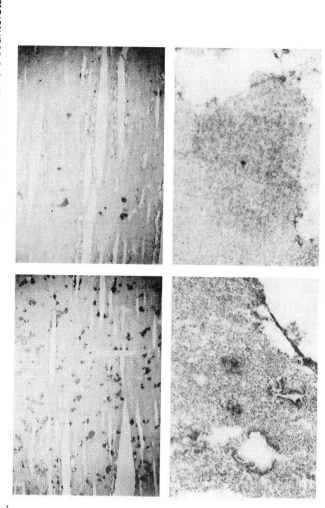

FIGURE 1. iNOS expression was deficient in mice with PCM. Tissue from BCG-infected CD1 mice with PCM (right panel) and those fed a normal diet (left panel) were studied for the expression of macrophage iNOS by immunohistochemical staining. Micrographs shown represent liver (top panel; 40 ×) and lung (bottom panel; 100 ×) tissues from animals harvested at day 5 and day 14 post-infection, respectively. OCT embedded fresh tissues were sectioned at 5-6 µm. A rabbit affinity purified polyclonal antibody against murine macrophage iNOS was applied at a dilution of 1:100 for 3-4 h. A conventional avidin-biotin complex method was performed using the ABC Vectastain Kit. Peroxidase-diaminobenzidine (DAB) method was used for colorization. The sections were counterstained with hematoxylin.

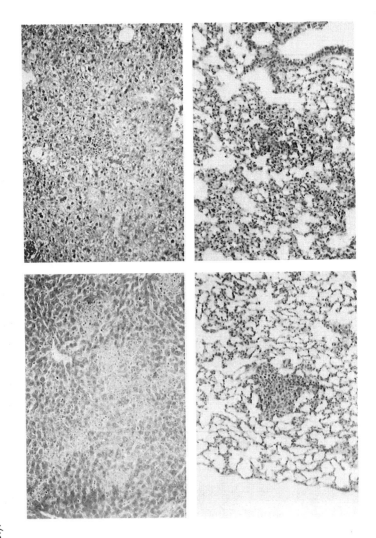

FIGURE 2. Granuloma formation was compromised in mice with PCM. Tissues from BCG-infected CD1 mice were studied after application of Hematoxylin and Eosin stain. Micrographs shown represent liver (top panel; 100×) and lung (bottom panel; 200×) sections of animals sacrificed 7 and 14 days post-infection, respectively. Mice fed 2% protein diet (right panel) exhibited poor granuloma formation compared to animals given a normal full-protein diet (left panel).

16

FIGURE 3. Bacillary burden was increased in mice with PCM. Tissues from BCG-infected CD1 mice were studied using the Kinyoun's acid fast stain. Micrographs shown represent liver sections (400×) obtained from animals 21 days post-infection. Bacillary burden of mice fed a protein-deficient diet (top panel) far exceeded that of animals given a normal diet (bottom panel). Examination of lung tissues showed similar results.

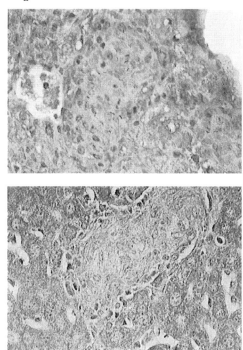

the mycobacteriocidal L-arginine-dependent cytotoxic pathway is deficient in protein calorie malnourished mice, particularly during the early non-immune phase of BCG infection when the antimycobacterial effect of RNI is deemed most critical for resistance against invading microbes.[21-23] Therefore, unrestricted bacterial growth in the early phase of infection secondary to compromised RNI production is likely to play a role in exacerbated disease progression observed in BCG-infected mice with PCM. Second, deficiency in granuloma formation, an immunological response generally considered critical in defense against mycobacterial infection, may have direct deleterious effect on disease outcome in protein calorie malnourished animals. Understanding the mechanisms by which iNOS expression and granuloma formation are compromised during mycobacterial infection in hosts with PCM is likely to help gain insight into the relationship between infection and malnutrition. Finally, our murine PCM model may afford an appropriate setting in which to examine the regulation of iNOS expression and the granulomatous reaction in tuberculosis.

Although it is generally accepted that PCM affects cellular immunity,[4,5] direct evidence of how malnutrition leads to increased risk of infections is lacking. The present study provides evidence that deficient expression of iNOS and poor granuloma formation may contribute, at least partially, to the increased susceptibility to BCG infection in mice with PCM. The significance of these findings in protein calorie malnourished mice infected with virulent *M. tuberculosis* is currently being examined.

REFERENCES

1. Rich, A. (1944). *The pathogenesis of tuberculosis*, Charles C. Thomas, Publisher, Springfield, Ill.

2. Bloom, B.R. and Murray, C.J.L. (1992). Tuberculosis: Commentary on a reemergent killer. Science 257:1055-1063.

3. Murray, C.J.L., Styblo, K., and Rouillon, A. (1990). Tuberculosis in developing countries: burden, intervention, and cost. Bull. Int. Union Tuberc. 65:2-24.

4. Chandra, R.K. (1991). Nutrition and Immunity: lessons from the past and new insights into the future. Am. J. Clin. Nutr. 53:1087-1101.

5. McMurray, D.N. (1994). Guinea pig model of tuberculosis. In *Tuberculosis. Pathogenesis, Protection, and Control*, Bloom, B.R. (ed.), ASM Press, Washington, DC., pp. 135-147.

6. Denis, M. (1991). Interferon-gamma-treated murine macrophages inhibit growth of tubercle bacilli via the generation of reactive nitrogen intermediates. Cell. Immunol. 132:150-157

7. Flesch, I.E.A. and Kaufmann, S.H.E. (1991). Mechanisms involved in mycobacterial growth inhibition by gamma interferon-activated bone marrow macrophages: role of reactive nitrogen intermediates. Infect. Immun. 59:3213-3218.

8. Chan, J. Xing, Y., Magliozzo, R.S., and Bloom, B.R. (1992). Killing of virulent *Mycobacterium tuberculosis* by reactive nitrogen intermediates produced by activated murine macrophages. J. Exp. Med. 175:1111-1122.

9. Ding, A.K. Nathan, C.F., and Stuehr, D.J. (1988). Release of reactive nitrogen intermediates and reactive oxygen intermediates from mouse peritoneal macrophages. J. Immunol. 141:2407-2412.

10. Stuehr, D.J. and Marietta, M.A. (1985). Mammalian nitrate biosynthesis: Mouse macrophages produce nitrite and nitrate in response to *Escherichia coli* lipopolysaccharide. Proc. Natl. Acad. Sci. USA. 82:7738-7742.

11. Roach, T.I.A., Barton, C.H., Chatterjee, D., and Blackwell, J.M. (1993). Macrophage activation: Lipoarabinomannan from avirulent and virulent strains of *Mycobacterium tuberculosis* differentially induces the early genes c-fos, KC, JE, and tumor necrosis factor-α. J. Immunol. 150:1886-1896.

12. Kamijo, R., Le, J., Shapiro, D., Havell, E.A., Huang, S., Auget, M., Bosland, M., and Vilcek, J. (1993). Mice that lack the interferon-γ receptor have profoundly altered responses to infection with Bacillus Calmette-Guerin and subsequent challenge with lipopolysaccharide. J. Exp. Med. 178:1435-1440.

13. Dalton, D.K., Pitts-Meek, S., Keshav, S., Figari, I.S., Bradley, A., and Stewart, T.A. (1993). Multiple defects of immune cell function in mice with disrupted interferon-gamma genes. Science 259:1739-1742.

14. Flynn, J.L., Chan, J., Trieboid, K.J., Dalton, D.K., Stewart, T.A., and Bloom, B.R. (1993). An essential role for interferon gamma in resistance to *Mycobacterium tuberculosis* infection. J. Exp. Med. 178:2249-2254.

15. Cooper, A.M., Dalton, D.K., Stewart, T.A., Griffin, J.P., Russell, D.G., and Orme, I.M. (1993). Disseminated tuberculosis in IFN-gamma gene-disrupted mice. J. Exp. Med. 178:2243-2248.

16. Kamijo, R., Harada, H., Matsuyama, T., Bosland, M., Gerecitano, J., Shapiro, D., Le, J., Koh, S.I., Kimura, T., Green, S.J., Mak, T.W., Taniguchi, T., and Vilcek, J. (1994). Requirement for transcription factor IRF-in NO synthase induction in macrophages. Science 263:1612-1615.

17. Chan, I., Tanaka, K., Carroll, D., Flynn, J.L, and Bloom, B.R. (1994). Effect of nitric oxide inhibitors on murine infection with *M. tuberculosis*. Submitted.

18. Granger, D.L., Hibbs, Jr., J.B., and Broadnax, L.M. (1991). Urinary nitrate excretion in relation to murine macrophage activation. Influence of dietary L-arginine and oral N^G-monomethyl-L-arginine. J. Immunol. 146:1294-1302.

19. Orme, I.M. and Collins, F.M. (1994). Mouse model in tuberculosis. In *Tuberculosis. Pathogenesis, Protection, and Control*, Bloom B.R. (ed.), ASM Press, Washington, DC., pp. 113-134.

20. Reynolds, J.V., Redmond, H.P., Ueno, N., Steigman, C., Zeigler, M.M., Daly, J.M., and Johnston, Jr., R.B. (1992). Impairment of macrophage activation and granuloma formation by protein deprivation in mice. Cell. Immunol. 139: 493-504.

21. Beckerman, K.P., Rogers, H.W., Corbett, J.A., Schreiber, R.D., McDaniel, M.L, and Unanue, E.R. (1993). Release of nitric oxide during the T cell-dependent pathway of macrophage activation. Its role in resistance to *Listeria monocytogenes*. J. Immunol. 150:888-895.

22. Tripp, C.S., Wolf, S.F., and Unanue, E.R. (1993). Interleukin 12 and tumor necrosis factor α are costimulators of interferon γ production by natural killer cells in severe combined immunodeficiency mice with listeriosis, and interleukin 10 is a physiologic antagonist. Proc. Natl. Acad. Sci. USA. 90:3725-3729.

23. Locksley, R.M. (1993). Interleukin 12 in host defense against microbial pathogens. Proc. Natl. Acad. Sci. USA 90:5879-5880.

Vitamin A Nutritional Status– Relationship to the Infection and the Antibody Response

A. Catharine Ross, PhD

Shortly after vitamin A (retinol and its biological derivatives) was first recognized as an essential nutrient, and well before its chemical nature was known, investigators implicated vitamin A in the differentiation of tissues and in protection against infections. In a now-classic study published by Wolbach and Howe in the mid-1920s, the characteristic changes in epithelial morphology that accompany vitamin A deficiency were first described (see reference 1). These investigators noted that the linings of the trachea, lungs, bladder, and several other organs that are normally composed of a single layer of ciliated, columnar or cuboidal cells with interspersed mucous-secreting goblet cells were markedly altered in vitamin A-deficient rats, becoming stratified, squamous and keratinized. They also commented on the atrophy of the thymus of severely vitamin A-deficient rats, as well as changes in some of the regional lymph nodes. A few years later, it was reported that vitamin A-

---

A. Catharine Ross, Department of Nutrition, Pennsylvania State University, University Park, PA.

Address correspondence to: A. Catharine Ross, PhD, Department of Nutrition, Pennsylvania State University, 126A Henderson Building, University Park, PA 16802.

[Haworth co-indexing entry note]: "Vitamin A Nutritional Status–Relationship to the Infection and the Antibody Response." Ross, Catharine A. Co-published simultaneously in *Journal of Nutritional Immunology* (The Haworth Medical Press, an imprint of The Haworth Press, Inc.) Vol. 5, No. 1, 1997, pp. 21-27; and: *Nutritional Abnormalities in Infectious Diseases: Effects on Tuberculosis and AIDS* (ed: Christopher E. Taylor) The Haworth Medical Press, an imprint of The Haworth Press, Inc., 1997, pp. 21-27. Single or multiple copies of this article are available for a fee from The Haworth Document Delivery Service [1-800-342-9678, 9:00 a.m. - 5:00 p.m. (EST). E-mail address: getinfo@haworth.com].

21

deficient rats often died with histopathologic evidence of infection, and referred to vitamin A as "the anti-infective agent." By the late 1960s when Scrimshaw and coworkers[2] reviewed the literature on nutrition and infection for the World Health Organization, they described the relationship between vitamin A deficiency and most infections, including tuberculosis, as synergistic.

Even at present, however, little specific information exists regarding the role of this essential nutrient in the response to tuberculosis and related infections. Based on the general functions of vitamin A in maintaining epithelial integrity, it is reasonable to postulate, *a priori*, that a deficiency of this nutrient may compromise either the host's resistance to infection or its ability to respond to infection. This presentation reviews briefly some of the recent advances in understanding the basic mechanisms of vitamin A's action; the role of specific proteins in transporting retinol and facilitating its metabolism and the effect of nutritional status and infection on these processes; and the results of epidemiological data and experiments designed to probe the requirement for vitamin A in protective immunity.

ADVANCES IN UNDERSTANDING THE BASIC FUNCTIONS OF VITAMIN A

Within the past decade, much has been learned regarding the fundamental mechanism of action of vitamin A in target tissues. It is clear that retinol (derived from dietary retinyl esters or from the metabolism of beta-carotene) serves as the precursor for two principal metabolites, retinal and retinoic acid, that are produced from retinol through intracellular oxidative metabolism. In the retina, 11-*cis*-retinaldehyde combines with the visual protein, opsin, to form rhodopsin which fulfills vitamin A's function in signal transduction during the visual cycle. In numerous tissues throughout the organism, retinoic acid, either as the all-*trans* or the 9-*cis* isomer, serves a broader role as the ligand for a family of nuclear retinoid receptors that are part of the steroid hormone/thyroid hormone superfamily of ligand-activated transcription factors. These retinoid-receptor complexes are capable of interactions with DNA in the regulatory regions of a diverse array of genes, and of combining with other nuclear proteins. Thus, retinoic acid performs the complex functions of vitamin A in regulating gene expression, the differentiation of cells, and the development of the organism.

ROLES OF SPECIFIC PROTEINS
IN VITAMIN A TRANSPORT AND METABOLISM

To be activated to retinoic acid, retinol must be delivered to target tissues and oxidized. The transport and metabolism of retinoids is now recognized to be intimately linked to their association with specific binding proteins. In plasma, retinol is bound in a 1:1 ratio to retinol-binding protein (RBP), a 21-kDa protein synthesized mainly in the liver and secreted as the RBP-retinol complex. RBP has a short half-life in plasma (~ 2 days) and thus continued protein synthesis is required to maintain a normal level of RBP in the circulation. At least three nutrient deficiencies are known to reduce plasma RBP and retinol levels: inadequate protein or inadequate energy compromise RBP synthesis, while inadequate retinol compromises the secretion of holo-RBP from the liver. Additionally, it has been shown that during acute infections, the plasma levels of retinol and RBP fall, presumably because RBP is regulated as a negative acute-phase protein. Thus, hypovitaminosis A is difficult to interpret because its etiology may include nutritional factors, inflammation or both. Indeed, it is possible that the combination of moderate vitamin A deficiency and infection may result in an acute, severe deficiency of retinol for delivery to peripheral tissues.

The cytoplasm of many types of cells contains one or more cellular retinoid-binding proteins. Several of these proteins participate in the metabolism of retinol, including esterification for storage and oxidation to form retinoic acid. Vitamin A deficiency may alter these processes by reducing (1) the saturation of the cellular binding proteins with their ligands; (2) the expression of the binding proteins; and (3) the activity of certain metabolic enzymes. As examples, the expression of cellular retinol-binding protein in the lung is regulated by retinoic acid and the processes of vitamin A storage and mobilization in liver appear to be decreased and increased, respectively, during vitamin A deficiency.

From these various results, it is thus reasonable to speculate that nutritional deficiencies of protein, energy, and vitamin A act alone or together through several pathways to adversely affect the transport of retinol to target tissues and its conversion to retinoic acid within tissues.

EPIDEMIOLOGICAL STUDIES OF THE CONSEQUENCES OF VITAMIN A DEFICIENCY IN YOUNG CHILDREN

Prior to the 1980s, public health interventions with vitamin A focused mainly on the prevention of xerophthalmia and nutritional blindness. Beginning with observational studies conducted by Sommer and colleagues[3] in the early 1980s in a rural area of Indonesia, data have accumulated that children with moderate vitamin A deficiency, as evidenced by mild xerophthalmia (a history of night blindness and corneal Bitôt's spots) are at a greater risk of death than children without xerophthalmia. A number of randomized intervention trials have now been conducted to determine whether supplementing young children in populations with vitamin A deficiency can significantly reduce mortality. Whereas there was a statistically significant reduction in mortality in several of these trials, in other trials no significant effect was detected. By the early 1990s, sufficient data had been collected for an overview and meta-analysis of the combined results. A review of these studies involving a meta-analysis of eight community-based studies of vitamin A supplementation in young children, conducted in areas of the world where vitamin A deficiency is still a public health problem, showed an overall reduction of 23% in the relative risk of mortality in children whose vitamin A status was improved.[4] This and other meta-analyses have included data from over 175,000 children in 8 independent studies and have shown a highly statistically significant ($P < 1 \times 10^{-9}$) effect of vitamin A. Although vitamin A was provided as a large-dose supplement at 4-6 month intervals in most of the trials, it was noted that a large dose is not required in order to observe a reduction in mortality because there was also a significant decrease in mortality in a study in which vitamin A was provided weekly in dietary amounts.[4]

In several of the mortality trials, a reduction in fever, pneumonia or diarrheal disease was reported. However, a consistent and specific effect of vitamin A on morbidity has been difficult to prove. Based on a field study designed to investigate morbidity in detail, Arthur et al. reported (reviewed in reference 4) that children in Ghana who were supplemented with vitamin A showed no difference in the incidence or duration of diarrhea and acute respiratory infections; however, the *severity* of infection, especially for diarrheal disease, was reduced in children given vitamin A. Hospital-based clinical trials in children with complicated measles have also supported the benefit of vitamin A in reducing measles-related morbidity and mortality.

Although the mechanism of vitamin A in reducing mortality or morbidity is not yet understood, it seems most likely that the effect of this vitamin is on the response to infection, probably acting through the immune system, rather than on the incidence of infection. Beaton et al.[4] concluded that vitamin A supplementation had no important effect on the incidence or duration of diarrheal and respiratory tract infections, although vitamin A did reduce severe complications and case mortality from pneumonia in the hospital-based study of measles infection.

VITAMIN A AND THE ANTIBODY RESPONSE TO INFECTION OR SPECIFIC ANTIGENS

A number of human and animal studies have been designed to evaluate the effects of vitamin A status on specific antibody responses. Semba et al.[5] reported a 2-fold higher serum anti-tetanus IgG concentration in Indonesian children who had been supplemented with vitamin A. In children with measles who received vitamin A, anti-measles IgG was significantly higher on day 8 of study. Experimental vitamin A deficiency and repletion in the rat, mouse or chick has been used by several investigators to evaluate the effects of vitamin A status on the response to experimental pathogens or antigens (see reference 1 for a detailed review). Generally, vitamin A deficiency has resulted in a low antibody response to T cell-dependent (TD) antigens or antigens that are known to be regulated by T cells (*type 2* antigens such as the capsular polysaccharides of *Streptococcus pneumoniae* and *Neisseria meningitidis*). In a comparative study of TD, *type 2* and *type 1* (lipopolysaccharide) antigens, vitamin A-deficient rats made very low antibody-specific responses to the TD antigens (tetanus toxoid and sheep red blood cells), similar to results for other TD protein antigens in mice and chicks, and low responses to the *type 2* capsular polysaccharide antigens, even before physical signs of vitamin A deficiency were apparent.[1,6] However, in contrast, the antibody response to *type 1* antigens (lipopolysaccharide antigens from *Pseudomonas aeruginosa* and *Serratia marcescens*) was normal, even after physical signs of vitamin A deficiency had developed. These data, together with normal or even elevated levels of total IgG, imply that antibody production *per se* is not limited by vitamin A deficiency but, rather, that *specific* responses that require T lymphocytes are reduced. Provision of retinol, *in vivo* and *in vitro*, rapidly reversed the low antibody responses.[1,3]

Despite little specific information on the response to BCG or active tuberculosis, these data on other immune responses suggest that vitamin A should be important both through its action in promoting the normal differentiation of mucosal cells, as related to the repair of injured epithelia, and through an effect on antibody production and protective immunity.

RETINOIDS AND IMMUNE STIMULATION

Whereas the studies above have focused on vitamin A deficiency and repletion, there is also evidence that vitamin A may, under some circumstances, stimulate immune responses even in vitamin A-sufficient animals or humans. Immune responses that have been reported to be increased following vitamin A administration include antibody production (adjuvant properties of retinoids), tumor immunity, expression of certain cell surface receptors, and functions of polymorphonuclear cells and phagocytes (see reference 1). Enhanced phagocytosis and clearance from blood have been reported for unrelated microbes (*Listeria*, *Candida*, and *Salmonella*) suggesting a nonspecific stimulation of clearing mechanisms by vitamin A. Vitamin A is also required for maintenance of a normal number of natural killer (NK) cells and normal cytotoxicity, and retinoic acid may stimulate NK cell cytotoxicity.[6]

Further investigations regarding the effect of vitamin A supplementation on the specific response to BCG vaccine and, especially on the response to active infection, are needed. It is likely that vitamin A status is an important determinant of the response to tuberculosis and related infections, based on knowledge gained from studies with other bacterial antigens and infectious diseases. Furthermore, we do not yet understand the cause of inflammation-induced hypovitaminosis A nor its consequences on the transport of retinol to peripheral tissues and the ability of the immune system to respond effectively to infection.

REFERENCE

1. Ross, A.C. and Hämmerling, U. (1994). Retinoids and the immune system. In: *The Retinoids: chemistry metabolism and medicine*, Sporn, M.B., Roberts, A.B., and Goodman, D.S. (eds.), Raven Press, NY, pg. 521-543.

2. Scrimshaw, N.S., Taylor, C.E., and Gordon, J.E. (1968). Interactions of nutrition and infection. WHO Monograph Series No. 57, World Health Organization, Geneva, Switzerland, pp. 60-329.

3. Sommer, A., Tarwotjo, I., Hussaini, G., and Susanto, D. (1983). Increased mortality in children with mild vitamin A deficiency. Lancet 2 (8350): 585-8.

4. Beaton, G.H., Martorell, R., Aronson, K.J., Edmonston, B., McCabe, G., Ross, A.C., and Harvey, B. (1993). Effectiveness of vitamin A supplementation in the control of young child morbidity and mortality in developing countries. ACC/SCN State-of-the-Art Series Nutrition Policy Discussion Paper No. 13, World Health Organization, Geneva.

5. Semba, R.D., Muhilal, Scott, A.L., Natadisastra, G., Wirasasmita, S., Mele, L., Ridwan, E., West, K.P., and Sommer, A. (1992). Depressed immune reponse to tetanus in children with vitamin A deficiency. J. Nutr. 122: 101-7.

6. Ross, A.C., Zhao, Z., Arora, D., Pasatiempo, A.M.G., Kinoshita, M., Gardner, E.M., Sri Kantha, S., and Taylor, C.E. (1993). Retinoids in specific and non-specific immunity: studies on antibody production and natural killer cells. In: *Retinoids progress in research and clinical applications*, Proceedings of the European Retinoids Research Conference, Livrea, M.A. and Packer, L. (eds.), Marcel Dekker, Inc., NY.

Modulation of Phagocyte Function by Nutrition in HIV-1 Infection

Steven D. Douglas, MD

Protein energy malnutrition (Kwashiorkor, Marasmus) remains a major world health problem. The main syndromes of severe infantile protein calorie malnutrition have been extensively studied from an immunologic perspective. The effects of malnutrition on immunologic and host defense mechanisms include effects on nonspecific factors such as skin and mucous membranes, acute phase reactants, complement activity, immunoglobulin levels, phagocyte function, and cell mediated immunity.[1] Malnutrition leads to altered function of the two major phagocytic cells, the neutrophil and mononuclear phagocyte.[1] These effects may be further altered by viral and/or bacterial infections. Furthermore, the influence of HIV-1 infection and tuberculosis on phagocyte function may further potentiate deficiencies in cell function.

Steven D. Douglas, Division of Allergy/Immunology, Children's Hospital, Philadelphia, PA.

Address correspondence to: Stephen D. Douglas, MD, Division of Allergy/Immunology, Children's Hospital, 34th Street & Civic Center Boulevard, Philadelphia, PA 19104-4399.

[Haworth co-indexing entry note]: "Modulation of Phagocyte Function by Nutrition in HIV-1 Infection." Douglas, Steven D. Co-published simultaneously in *Journal of Nutritional Immunology* (The Haworth Medical Press, an imprint of The Haworth Press, Inc.) Vol. 5, No. 1, 1997, pp. 29-32; and: *Nutritional Abnormalities in Infectious Diseases: Effects on Tuberculosis and AIDS* (ed: Christopher E. Taylor) The Haworth Medical Press, an imprint of The Haworth Press, Inc., 1997, pp. 29-32. Single or multiple copies of this article are available for a fee from The Haworth Document Delivery Service [1-800-342-9678, 9:00 a.m. - 5:00 p.m. (EST). E-mail address: getinfo@haworth.com].

29

PHAGOCYTE FUNCTION IN MALNUTRITION IN HUMANS AND IN EXPERIMENTAL ANIMALS

A complex series of events are involved in phagocytic function. These include: adherence, chemotaxis, opsonization and engulfment, and post-phagocytic events, which include phagocytic vacuole formation, lysosome-phagosome fusion, metabolic events, including an oxidative burst, and production of reactive oxygen intermediates, and, in some instances, the production of nitric oxide and other nitrogen intermediates by cytokine activated cells.

NEUTROPHIL IN MALNUTRITION

The neutrophil is the initial cell which responds in acute inflammation. Adhesion to endothelium is a requisite for cell migration and locomotion and involves events which involve several adhesion molecules. Studies of animal models and patients with protein malnutrition have shown modulation of adherence, decreased random and directed movement, and decreased microbicidal activity.[1] Our laboratory has investigated a newborn rat model of postnatal malnutrition in the Wistar rat, using either a normal 24% protein or an isocaloric 2.5% protein diet. The malnutrition produced was for calories and protein because of the decreased appetite of the animals. Following 21 days gestation, the mothers on the restriction delivered pups that were small for gestational age compared to normally nourished pups. In this newborn rat model,[2] we have observed diminished weight gain, diminished protein and albumin. In this system, neutrophil adherence chemotaxis and microbicidal activity for *Staphylococcus aureus* were observed to be diminished; hydrogen peroxide was enhanced. These defects in phagocyte function, although the mechanism is unknown, contribute to increased susceptibility to infection in the neonate.[1,2]

MONONUCLEAR PHAGOCYTE IN MALNUTRITION

Studies of the mononuclear phagocyte in malnutrition thus far have shown evidence in the decrease in microbicidal and viricidal activity. Fibronectin levels in the serum, a secretory product of mononuclear phagocytes, are decreased in infants with protein calorie malnutrition, and increase to greater than normal values following nutritional support.[3]

MONOCYTE MACROPHAGES
IN HIV-1 AND TUBERCULOSIS

The macrophage is a major target cell infected by HIV-1.[4] Strains of HIV have varying degrees of monocyte/macrophage tropism.[4] Macrophage products, particularly cytokines may up and down regulate viral infectivity. The relationship between cytokines and infectivity of phagocytes has long been of considerable interest. In 1918, Ishigami[5] demonstrated that opsonic indices were reduced in macrophages incubated with tubercle bacilli intraperitoneally and that glucose and adrenaline further inhibited the opsonic index. This is the first report of a possible relationship between stress and tuberculosis.[5] In *in vitro* experiments, Ellner et al.[6,7] demonstrated that IL2, IL4, 1,25 dihydroxy vitamin D3, GM-CSF (TNF-α) and interferon-γ are activating cytokines for *Mycobacterium avium* and in some instances *Mycobacterium tuberculosis*. In contrast, IL1, IL3, IL6, IL10, TGF-β and PGE2 are deactivating cytokines. In slim disease associated with AIDS, serum levels of interleukin-1β, tumor necrosis factor α, interleukin 6, and acute phase proteins[8] are considerably elevated in contrast to other HIV-infected patients. In dually infected hosts[6,7] there is an inverse relationship between mycobacterial virulence and the capacity of the organism to produce protective cytokines in the host. In particular, decrease in interferon-γ is associated with increased progressive post-primary disease, and in fact a recent clinical trial of interferon-γ has shown improvement in *Mycobacterium avium* infection.[9] The situation is further complicated by effects of malnutrition and the fact that TNF-α may increase HIV expression.

Thus, relationships between malnutrition, tuberculosis, and HIV-1 infection have a panoply of effects on the phagocytes. These effects are interactive and may potentiate clinical disease. The design of various interventions, including cytokine and anti-cytokine therapy must consider these important interactions.

REFERENCES

1. Harris, M.C. and Douglas, S.D. (1990). Nutritional influence on neonatal infections in animal models and man. Annals of the New York Academy of Science–Micronutrients and Immune functions. 587:246-256.

2. Harris, M.C., Douglas, S.D., Chiang, J.L., Ziegler, M.M., Gerdes, J.S., and Polin, R.A. (1987). Diminished polymorphonuclear leukocyte adherence and chemotaxis following protein-calorie malnutrition in newborn rats. Pediatr. Res. 21:542-546.

3. Yoder, M.C., Anderson, D.C., Gopalakrishna, G.S., Douglas, S.D., and Polin, R.A. (1987). Comparison of serum fibronectin, prealbumin and albumin concentrations during nutritional repletion in protein-calorie malnourished infants. J. Pediatr. Gastroenterol. Nutr. 6:84-88.

4. Ho, W-Z, Cherukuri, R., and Douglas, S.D. (1994). The macrophage and HIV-1. In: *Macrophage-Pathogen Interactions*, Marcel Dekker, Inc. (ed. by Zwilling, B.S. and Eisenstein, T.K.) pp. 569-587.

5. Ishigami, T. (1918-1919). The influence of psychic acts on the progress of pulmonary tuberculosis. American Review of Tuberculosis. 2:470-487.

6. Wallis, R.S. and Ellner, J.J. (1994). Cytokines and tuberculosis. I. Leukocyte Biol. 55:676-681.

7. Shiratsuchi, H., Johnson, J.L., Toossi, Z., and Ellner, J.J. (1994). Modulation of the effector function of human monocytes for *Mycobacterium avium* by human immunodeficiency virus-I envelope glycoprotein gp120. J. Clin. Invest. 93:885-891.

8. Belec, L, Meillet, D., Hernvann, A., Gresenguet, G., and Gherardi, R. (1994). Differential elevation of circulating interleukin-1b, tumor necrosis factor alpha, and interleukin-6 in AIDS-associated cachectic states. Clin. Diagn. Lab. Immunol. 1:117-120.

9. Holland, S.M., Eisenstein, E.M., Kuhns, D.B., Turner, M.L., Fleisher, T.A., Strober, W., and Gallin, J.I. (1994). Treatment of refractory disseminated nontuberculous mycobacterial infection with interferon gamma. N. Engl. J. Med. 330:1348-1355.

Malnutrition as a Co-Factor
in HIV Disease

Susanna Cunningham-Rundles, PhD
Lenora M. Noroski, MD
Joseph S. Cervia, MD

Malnutrition has been recognized as a major cause of immune deficiency long before the appearance of the Human Immunodeficiency Virus, HIV.[1] While the general importance of nutritional status in the control of infectious diseases in general is well known, the potential role of nutrition as a cofactor in HIV infection has not been established. Although weight loss, malabsorption, trace element deficiency, and unexplained changes in metabolism may lead to a wasting syndrome in HIV infected persons, the possibility that nutrient deficiency represents an etiologic factor in HIV progression has remained controversial.[2]

A few studies have suggested that nutrient deficiency may occur early during the asymptomatic phase of HIV infection in adults.[3,4]

Susanna Cunningham-Rundles is affiliated with the Department of Pediatrics, New York Hospital-Cornell University Medical Center. Lenora M. Noroski is affiliated with the Department of Pediatrics, Baylor College, Waco, TX. Joseph S. Cervia is affiliated with the Department of Pediatrics, Division of Infectious Diseases, Cornell Medical College, New York, NY.

Address correspondence to Susanna Cunningham-Rundles, PhD, Department of Pediatrics, New York Hospital-Cornell University Medical Center, 525 E. 68th Street, New York, NY 10021-4805.

[Haworth co-indexing entry note]: "Malnutrition as a Co-Factor in HIV Disease." Cunningham-Rundles, Susanna, Lenora M. Noroski, and Joseph S. Cervia. Co-published simultaneously in *Journal of Nutritional Immunology* (The Haworth Medical Press, an imprint of The Haworth Press, Inc.) Vol. 5, No. 1, 1997, pp. 33-38; and: *Nutritional Abnormalities in Infectious Diseases: Effects on Tuberculosis and AIDS* (ed: Christopher E. Taylor) The Haworth Medical Press, an imprint of The Haworth Press, Inc., 1997, pp. 33-38. Single or multiple copies of this article are available for a fee from The Haworth Document Delivery Service [1-800-342-9678, 9:00 a.m. - 5:00 p.m. (EST). E-mail address: getinfo@haworth.com].

Because HIV triggers cytokine activation,[5] which may produce a hypermetabolic state leading to altered food intake, interference with absorption, and cause reactivation of viral infections other than HIV, it seems possible that there may be a critical interaction between nutrients and HIV at several levels. A key regulator of these effects appears to be Tumor Necrosis Factor α, TNFα. This cytokine, also referred to as cachectin is known to mediate a wasting syndrome in chronic infection and cancer as well as enhance wound healing and destroy tumors when secreted locally (at low levels).[6] Infusion of TNFα appears to produce pathological sequelae that mimic infection.[7] Among HIV+ children, Mintz et al. have found that TNFα production was increased in association with progressive encephalopathy.[8] TNFα has the ability to upregulate HIV. In addition, TNFα and Interleukin 6, IL-6, which increase in HIV infection appear to activate HIV harbored as proviral DNA by activating replication.[9]

In pediatric HIV infection, the need for nutritional supplementation has been identified as a potential issue in clinical management;[10] however, there have been no studies done to address such basic issues in order to determine whether or not defined changes in nutritive status may precede specific decline in CD_4+ T cell number or T cell function, or precede evidence of clinical progression of the disease. The postnatal period is a time of particular sensitivity to nutrient deprivation. Before the appearance of HIV, breast milk was the chief means whereby infants in compromised environments were able to survive endemic infections and chronic nutrient deficits.[11] The importance of breast milk in the neonatal period has been widely recognized for all infants; however, breast milk must be withheld when the mother is HIV infected. Nutrient deficiency may be critically important in a unique way in the HIV+ child and even potentially trigger events leading to a transition between clinical latency and overt HIV disease. We have recently begun to assess the relationship between nutrient imbalance, immune status, and susceptibility to opportunistic infections, particularly *Pneumocystis carinii* pneumonia and mycobacterial infections, in children congenitally exposed to HIV. About one third of HIV+ children in our clinic, show poor growth and development, and in a subset of these cases, the children are otherwise asymptomatic. In contrast, adults with HIV infection demonstrate significant malnutrition mainly in advanced disease. While the progress of HIV infection in children is often faster than in adults, this may occur in the absence of significant decline in CD_4+ T cell number suggesting that other factors, including nutrient deficiency which may trigger events in a unique way in the congenitally HIV+ infected infant, may also be critically important.

In the current studies we carried out immune analysis of more than 70 babies ($\leq$ 12 months at the time of the first study) born to HIV+ mothers. We observed that 45% of the babies were ultimately found to be seroreverters, and 51% were infected. When CD_4+T cell levels at the first study were analyzed retrospectively, the seroreverting infants were found to have T cell levels comparable to those of age-matched infants not exposed to HIV and greater than those from HIV infected infants (p < 0.001). Using normal (greater than 1) compared to abnormal (less than 1) CD_4/CD_8 ratio as a means of classification, we found that there were 22 infants (GROUP B) with inverted CD_4/CD_8 ratios and 17 infants with normal CD_4/CD_8 (GROUP A) ratios. There was a significant difference between those with a normal CD_4/CD_8 ratio (A) and those with a reversed CD_4/CD_8 ratio (B) with respect to CD_4+ T cell percentage (p < 0.001). The Group A infants could not be positively identified as HIV infected individuals at the time of first study and did not meet criteria for prophylaxis against opportunistic infection. However, more than half of the infants developed HIV associated symptoms before the demonstration of a significant loss of percent CD_4+ T cells. These findings highlight a key distinction from the T cell levels in HIV positive adults. Here, the decrease in CD_4 precedes development of opportunistic infection and suggest that alteration in immune function specific to congenital HIV infection and preceding overt CD_4+ T cell loss might be fundamental to the development of HIV related symptoms. It is not unreasonable to assume that the effect of subtle regional HIV replication would have a proportionately greater effect on the growing infant if this viral activity triggered malabsorption and malnutrition. The clinical state of *failure-to-thrive* is a well known phenomenon in pediatrics. Frequently, the cause is often not convincingly established although it is generally assumed that unidentified viral infection or that perhaps the combination of normal immaturity, chance exposure to a common virus, and nutrient insufficiency is the basis of the syndrome.

In parallel with the AIDS epidemic, infection with *Mycobacterium tuberculosis* has re-emerged as a significant pathogen in the United States. Susceptibility to *M. tuberculosis* is known to be associated with malnutrition. Furthermore, the HIV infected host is significantly more vulnerable to this pathogen.[12] Mycobacterial infections, specifically with normally nonpathogenic species which are opportunistic in the immunocompromised host, are a serious complication of HIV infection in children. During the past five years we observed that out of 15 HIV+ children who were also culture positive for mycobacterial infections (2 with *M. tuberculosis*, and 13 with *M. avium* complex), none remain alive. In our clinic we have found, based on culture positive cases, that *M. tuberculosis* infections have increased 2 fold in each of three successive five year intervals since 1975-1980. This is likely to be an underestimation of the actual incidence, since awareness of this pathogen has not been widespread. Because HIV status was not sought in children presenting with *M. tuberculosis* infections, co-infection rate was not established.

We have initiated an evaluation of nutritional parameters, immune function, and susceptibility to infection, with particular reference to mycobacterial infection in the HIV+ child in comparison with non-HIV+ children infected with *M. tuberculosis* or other mycobacterial infections. Preliminary data are presented here. Of 10 babies less than one year of age, who had been congenitally exposed to HIV and were being evaluated for possible developmental delay, 5 were found to have T cell subset ratio within normal range and 5 had abnormal subset ratios. As shown in Table 1, all babies with abnormal T cell subsets had evidence of growth abnormality, but there was no relationship between the degree of T cell deficit, as measured by absolute CD_4 T cell number and the degree of growth abnormality. Of the 4 babies with normal T cell subset ratios, 2 had marked growth delay and 2 did not. Preliminary data suggest that growth rate rather than length or height alone may be a better reflection of the effect of HIV, since some children who do not fall below the 5th percentile for height and weight alone are clearly and consistently below the 5th percentile for velocity of growth.

TABLE 1. HIV Exposure and Growth

Case	Age at Entry	CD$_4$/CD$_8$ Ratio 1st Study	Absolute CD$_4$ number	Growth*
#1	11 months	Abnormal	63	Rate*
#2	10 months	Abnormal	821	Rate*
#3	8 months	Abnormal	944	Length*
#4	1 month	Abnormal	2025	Length*
#5	2 weeks	Abnormal	826	Length*
#6	1 month	Normal	3232	Length*
#7	1 month	Normal	5246	Head*
#8	1 month	Normal	3818	Head, Rate*
#9	1 month	Normal	2213	Length*
#10	3 months	Normal	4284	Normal

* At 5th percentile or less

In contrast, studies conducted during the past six months on 6 children who were culture positive for *M. tuberculosis* but negative for HIV infection, indicate that weight loss has been observed only during febrile episodes and that overt malnutrition has not been seen. T cell subset abnormalities were observed in some of the children, but these changes were transient, and resolved with treatment. Both weight loss and T cell abnormalities in this setting are therefore likely to be secondary to cytokine activation in these previously well children.

Thus, our current ongoing studies suggest that HIV infection may have a direct effect on nutrient status and growth in the exposed infant, separately from that developing as a consequence of clinically significant opportunistic infection arising from a decline in CD4+ T cell level. Thus, malnutrition in the HIV infected host may affect susceptibility to opportunistic and environmental infections and therefore be a cofactor in progression of disease. Since infection with *M. tuberculosis* is also linked to malnutrition, future efforts to identify links and mechanisms could provide new direction to the study of the interactions among nutrition, immunity, and host defense against infection.

REFERENCES

1. Curningham-Rundles, S. (1981). Effect of nutritional status on immunological function. Am. J. Clin. Nutr., 35:1202-1210.

2. Editorial. (1991). Nutrition and HIV. Lancet 338:860.

3. Melchior, J.D., Salmon, D., Rigaud, D., Shigenaga, Jenson, P., and Feingold, K.R. (1991). Resting energy expenditure is increased in stable, malnourished HIV- infected patients. Am. J. Clin. Nutr. 53:437-441.

4. Grunfeld, C., Pang, M., Shimizu, L., Shigenaga, J.K., Jensin, P., and Feingold, K.R. (1992). Resting energy expenditure, calorie intake, and short term weight change in human immunodeficiency virus infection and the acquired immunodeficiency syndrome. Am. J. Clin. Nutr. 55:455-460.

5. Scott Algara, D., Vuiller, T., Marasescu, M., de Saint Martin, J., and Dighiero, G. (1991). Serum levels of IL-2, IL-Iα, TNF-α and soluble receptor of IL-2 in HIV-infected patients. AIDS Research and Human Retro. 7:381-386.

6. Moldawer, L.L. and Lowry, S.F. (1993). Interactions between cytokine production and inflammation: implications for therapies aimed at modulating the host defense to infection. In: *Nutrient Modulation of Immune Response*, Cunningham-Rundles, S. (ed.), Marcel Dekker, Inc., p. 511.

7. Tracey, K.J., Beulter, B., Lowry, S.F., Merry Weather, J., Volpe, S., Milsark, I.W., Hariri, R.I., Fahey, T.J., Zentella, A., Albert, J.D., Shires, G.T., and Cerami, A. (1986). Shock and tissue injury induced by recombinant human cachectin. Science 234:470-474.

8. Mintz, M., Rapaport, R., Oleske, J.M., Connor, E.M., Koenigsberger, M.R., Denny, T., and Epstein, L.G. (1989). Elevated serum levels of tumor necrosis factor are associated with progressive encephalopathy in children with acquired immunodeficiency syndrome. Am. J. Dis. Child. 143:771-774.

9. Poli, G., Kinter, A., Justement, J.S., Kenrl, J.H., Bressler, P., Stanley, S., and Fauci, A. (1990). Tumor necrosis factor α functions in an autocrine manner in the induction of human immunodeficiency virus expression. Proc. Natl. Acad. Sci. 87:782-785.

10. Nicholas, S.W., Leung, J., and Fennoy I. (1991). Guidelines for nutritional support of HIV infected children. I. Pediatr. 119:S59-62.

11. Hanson, L.A., Adlerberth, I., Carlsson, B.U.M., Hahn Zoric, M., Jalil, F., Mellander, L., Robertson, D.M., and Zaman, S. (1993). Human milk antibodies and their importance for the infant. In: *Nutrient Modulation of Immune Response*, Cunningham-Rundles, S. (ed.), Marcel Dekker, Inc. p. 525.

12. Collins, F.M. (1989). Mycobacterial disease, immunosuppression, and acquired immunodeficiency syndrome. Clin. Microbiol. Rev. 2: 360-377.

Clinical Aspects of Nutrition in Tuberculosis

Gwen A. Huitt, MD

The word "consumption" has long been used to describe the process by which individuals with tuberculosis undergo a transformation from robust, healthy individuals, into frail and emaciated shadows of themselves. Indeed, the ancient Greeks called the condition "phthisis" which translated into "I am wasting." This accurately describes the disturbance that occurs when disease caused by *Mycobacterium tuberculosis* (MTB) creates a physiologic environment where catabolism grossly exceeds anabolism. The state of catabolism sets the stage for gradual caloric deficits and ultimately leads to a state of clinical malnutrition.[1] It has been our experience at the National Jewish Center for Immunology and Respiratory Medicine (NJC), that most patients are clinically malnourished upon admission to our facility. Of the last 63 patients treated at NJC for chronic drug-resistant tuberculosis, 75% had some degree of malnutrition. Of those, 42% were found to be either moderately or severely malnourished based on Diagnosis Related Group (DRG) criteria (unpublished data). Therefore, our treatment goals include

Gwen A. Huitt, Division of Infectious Diseases, National Jewish Center for Immunology & Respiratory Medicine, Denver, CO.

Address correspondence to: Gwen A. Huitt, MD, Division of Infectious Diseases, National Jewish Center for Immunology & Respiratory Medicine, 1400 Jackson Avenue, Denver, CO 80406.

[Haworth co-indexing entry note]: "Clinical Aspects of Nutrition in Tuberculosis." Huitt, Gwen A. Co-published simultaneously in *Journal of Nutritional Immunology* (The Haworth Medical Press, an imprint of The Haworth Press, Inc.) Vol. 5, No. 1, 1997, pp. 39-44; and: *Nutritional Abnormalities in Infectious Diseases: Effects on Tuberculosis and AIDS* (ed: Christopher E. Taylor) The Haworth Medical Press, an imprint of The Haworth Press, Inc., 1997, pp. 39-44. Single or multiple copies of this article are available for a fee from The Haworth Document Delivery Service [1-800-342-9678, 9:00 a.m. - 5:00 p.m. (EST). E-mail address: getinfo@haworth.com].

appropriate antituberculous chemotherapy as well as nutritional optimization.

There are many factors that contribute to the catabolic state and malnutrition in patients with tuberculosis. Most believe that it is elevated levels of tumor necrosis factor or "cachexin" that produces clinical signs and symptoms of fever, anorexia, and weight loss. In addition, patients with tuberculosis experience profound fatigue, which makes it extremely difficult to prepare or even consume a meal. Furthermore, sputum from tuberculous lungs often has a characteristic foul taste and odor which is quite noticeable to the patient, resulting in distorted taste (dysgeusia) and diminished desire to eat.

Many of the medications used to treat MTB infections can cause significant gastrointestinal side effects. A few of the more common examples are listed as follows: *INH/Rifampin* causes nausea/vomiting, anorexia, and hepatitis; *Ethionamide* causes nausea and vomiting, unusual odors to foods (particularly with meat), metallic taste, anorexia, endocrine disorders such as hypothyroidism; *PAS* causes nausea and vomiting, anorexia, diarrhea, endocrine disorders (particularly if patient is also taking ethionamide); *Ofloxacin/Ciprofloxacin* causes anorexia, hepatitis, and anxiety; and *Clarithromycin* causes nausea and metallic taste.

The gastrointestinal side effects of these medications have a profound impact on a patient's ability to consume sufficient calories. We have found that dyspepsia (i.e., bloating, nausea, heartburn) is predictable when ethionamide and PAS are administered together or individually within a medical regimen. Unfortunately, this may be unavoidable when drug susceptibilities dictate that these drugs must be used, particularly when administered simultaneously. To help alleviate the dyspepsia, we currently administer metoclopromide, 10 mg orally, thirty minutes prior to medication doses (either BID or TID). Antacids such as Maalox® and Mylanta® may be used to minimize dyspepsia, however, these compounds may cause diarrhea if consumed too frequently. It is also important to remember that both of these compounds contain aluminum which has been shown to significantly interfere with absorption of rifampin and the quinolones. Both rifampin and the quinolones bind divalent and trivalent cations, significantly lowering the serum drug concentration of these medications. Patients must avoid compounds containing iron, calcium, magnesium, and aluminum within 2 hours of ingesting these medications.[2]

Diarrhea is a common occurrence in patients who are taking PAS. The new, granule formulation has significantly diminished this problem, however, many patients continue to have difficulties. It is not uncommon for a patient to experience diarrhea approximately 3-5 days after PAS has been initiated. This is usually self-limited, and can be controlled easily with administration of loperamide 2 mg after each loose stool, not to exceed 12 mg per day. The diarrhea will usually resolve within a week. It is also important to explain to the patient that the quality of their stool will likely change while taking PAS, and that a "soft" stool is quite normal. Also, explain to patients that they may see the cellulose casings of the PAS granules in their stool. This is normal and it does not indicate malabsorption of the medication.

As noted, dysosmia (alteration in the sense of smell) and dysgeusia (alteration in the sense of taste) are common side effects associated with many medications administered for the treatment of mycobacterial infections. Most notable is clarithromycin. This drug is rarely used in treatment regimens for infections due to *M. tuberculosis*, but is commonly used to treat mycobacterial infections other than tuberculosis. Patients often complain of a persistent metallic taste as well as a significantly altered sense of taste when taking this medication. We have found that the unpleasant taste can be minimized by regular use of strong mints or candies. Also, if a patient finds that food odors are offensive, removing the cover from the plate (in hospitalized patients) before taking food into the room will help dissipate food associated odors. If a patient is at home, have the patient eat in a room other than the kitchen so they will not be subjected to the odors associated with food preparation.

Cultural tastes play a central role in providing adequate nutrition. NJC, as a worldwide referral center, typically has a patient population that is composed of many ethnic and cultural backgrounds. We have found that it is imperative to assess patients' food likes and dislikes upon admission to provide them with acceptable meal patterns. Our dietitians take a history that includes daily caloric intake as well as the types and amount of food that a patient normally consumes. Many patients consume only ethnic foods and we often enlist the help of family members to bring in requested foods. We also ask our dietary department to assist us in providing the special diet needs for our patients.

When these measures have been implemented and the patient continues to have diminished appetite, we will consider adding an appetite stimulant such as megestrol acetate.[3] We have found that starting a patient at a dose of 80 mg three times a day (TID) and increasing to a maximum of 160 mg TID will often promote significant improvement in caloric intake. We discontinue the megestrol after 3-4 weeks if the patient does not show any significant improvement in appetite.

Some patients are too ill to eat. For others, we are attempting to prepare them for surgical resection of badly damaged lung tissue in the near future.[4] In these cases, we commonly add total parenteral nutrition (TPN) and/or enteral feeding to optimize nutrition. We only use peripheral TPN on a temporary basis, i.e., 1-2 weeks.[5] Enteral feeding, however, is employed for many weeks or months. In these cases we place either nasogastric or PEG feeding tubes to make the process more comfortable and less burdensome for the patient.

Most patients are unaware of the basics of good nutrition, and evaluation by a registered dietician is a very valuable tool in helping both the physician and the patient manage their illness. At NJC each patient is followed by a registered dietician throughout their hospitalization. The initial evaluation consists of a detailed nutritional assessment. This objectively identifies high risk patients using a systematic method that includes: (1) medical history, (2) diet history (typical meal pattern, food preferences, food frequency), (3) anthropometrics, (4) biochemical parameters (albumin, prealbumin, transferrin, hematocrit, nitrogen balance), and (5) nutritional requirements (energy and protein needs). Using these parameters, a care plan and nutritional goals are established for each patient.

Small, frequent meals are usually better tolerated than conventional, large three-times-a-day meals. Morning and evening snacks, as well as liquid protein supplements such as Ensure®, Sustacal®, and Carnation Instant Breakfast® are important additions to regularly scheduled meals. Fruits and vegetables are important sources of vitamins and minerals that are commonly lacking in the diet of a patient with tuberculosis. Many antimycobacterial medications may actually cause vitamin deficiencies. PAS may cause malabsorption of vitamin B_{12} and fat soluble vitamins. Cycloserine and INH are both vitamin B_6 antagonists. Aminoglycosides promote renal wasting of potassium and magnesium. INH also causes a decrease in calcium absorption. Mild zinc deficiency likely contributes to the anemia and lethargy present in tuberculosis. Hence, we believe that it is very important that persons being treated for tuberculosis receive multivitamin supplements.

Malabsorption of antimycobacterial antibiotics is recognized to occur in many patients.[6-8] At NJC we routinely measure serum drug levels and utilize this pharmacological data to maximize medical therapy. It has been noted that patients with HIV and/or AIDS may significantly malabsorb these antibiotics, and inadequate therapy or drug resistance may result. We advocate the use of serum drug levels when managing any patient with a mycobacterial infection that the clinician suspects of malabsorption.

Thus, malnutrition has been noted to both precede and occur simultaneously with disease caused by *M. tuberculosis*. There are many factors responsible for the protein wasting including: (1) activation of the immune system with increased production of cytokines including TNF that promotes catabolism; (2) disease associated fever, cough, and anorexia; (3) medication induced anorexia, dyspepsia, and dysgeusia; and (4) malabsorption of vital nutrients and medications. There are many interventions available to clinicians, health care workers, and patients to help combat the myriad of problems encountered when treating nutritional difficulties caused by *M. tuberculosis*.

REFERENCES

1. McMurray D.N. and Bartow R.A. (1992). Immunosuppression and alteration of resistance to pulmonary tuberculosis in guinea pigs by protein undernutrition. I. Nutr. [122(3 suppl)]:38-43.

2. Peloquin, C.A. (1991). Antituberculosis drugs: Pharmacokinetics. In: *Drug susceptibility in the chemotherapy of mycobacterial infections*, Heifits L.B. (ed.), Boca Raton, FL, CRC Press, pp. 59-88.

3. Tchekmedyian N., Tait, N., Moody, M., and Aisner, J. (1987). High-dose megestrol acetate. JAMA 257:1195-1198.

4. Windsor J.A. and Hill, G.L. (1988). Weight loss with physiologic impairment: a basic indicator of surgical risk. Ann. Surg. 207:290-296.

5. Detsky, A.S. (1991). Parenteral nutrition: is it helpful? N. Engl. J. Med. 325:573-575.

6. Scalcini, M., Occenac, R., Manfreda, J., and Long, R. (1991). Pulmonary tuberculosis, human innnunodeficiency virus type-1 and malnutrition. Bull. Int. Union. Tuberc. Lung. Dis. 66:37-41.

7. Peloquin, C., Nitta, A., Burman, W., Brudney, K., McGuinness, M., Miranda-Massari, J., and Gerena, G. (1994). Incidence of low tuberculosis drug concentrations in AIDS patients. Abstract 34th Interscience Conference on Antimicrobial Agents and Chemotherapy, Orlando, FL, October 4-7.

8. Gordon, S.M., Horsburgh, C.R., Peloquin, C.A., Havlik, J.A., Metchock, B., Heifets, L., McGowan, J.E., and Thompson, S. (1993). Low serum levels of oral antimycobacterial agents in patients with disseminated *Mycobacterium avium* complex diseases. J Infect Dis. 168:1559-62.

Malnutrition and AIDS in the Developing World

Gerald T. Keusch, MD

EVIDENCE FOR MALNUTRITION

The initial recognition of AIDS occurred in Uganda in the late 1970's when previously healthy young men developed a new, recognizable, progressive, fatal wasting syndrome of unknown etiology, generally associated with chronic diarrhea, anorexia, and fever. This was called SLIM disease by the local population. Later, after HIV was discovered and a diagnostic serological test was developed, patients with SLIM disease were found to be HIV infected. In an earlier era, similar wasting associated with fever, cough, hemoptysis, and progressive respiratory impairment, ultimately shown to be due to *Mycobacterium tuberculosis*, was called consumption, as the host literally consumed his/her own body.

Studies of body composition carried out in the U.S. and Europe have elucidated several critical aspects of AIDS wasting syndrome. First, there is a progressive depletion of both body fat-free mass as well as fat mass, with the former predominating in males and, often

Gerald T. Keusch, Professor of Medicine and Chief, Division of Geographic Medicine and Infectious Diseases, New England Medical Center, Boston, MA.

Address correspondence to: Gerald T. Keusch, MD, Tufts University Medical School, 750 Washington Street, 5th Floor, Boston, MA 02111 USA.

[Haworth co-indexing entry note]: "Malnutrition and AIDS in the Developing World." Keusch, Gerald T. Co-published simultaneously in *Journal of Nutritional Immunology* (The Haworth Medical Press, an imprint of The Haworth Press, Inc.) Vol. 5, No. 1, 1997, pp. 45-50; and: *Nutritional Abnormalities in Infectious Diseases: Effects on Tuberculosis and AIDS* (ed: Christopher E. Taylor) The Haworth Medical Press, an imprint of The Haworth Press, Inc., 1997, pp. 45-50. Single or multiple copies of this article are available for a fee from The Haworth Document Delivery Service [1-800-342-9678, 9:00 a.m. - 5:00 p.m. (EST). E-mail address: getinfo@haworth.com].

the latter in females. Second, there is an increase in resting energy expenditure, which increases still further in the presence of infection. Third, there is a relative increase in body water, so that apparent weight loss is mitigated as the loss of body cell mass proceeds. Assessment of weight does not, therefore, detect the changes in body composition that occur early in the course of HIV infection. The causes are multifactorial and these vary during disease progression. These may be grouped into three categories, first, decreased nutrient intake (anorexia, dysphagia, esophageal or bowel obstruction, weakness/lethargy), second, malabsorption (structural abnormalities, specific gut infections, AIDS enteropathy, small bowel overgrowth syndrome), and third, metabolic disturbances (tissue catabolism, increased energy expenditure, futile metabolic cycles, altered patterns of anabolism, cytokine driven metabolic changes). Whatever the cause, loss of cell mass is an independent predictor of death in AIDS patients. In patients followed serially, extrapolated cell mass at death was reduced to approximately 55% of normal, a figure in common estimated body cell mass in patients dying of starvation or associated with cancer cachexia.[1]

Methods to assess body composition include anthropometry, the measurement of weight, height, skinfold thickness in various locations, and limb circumference, as well as derived normalized indices such as body cell mass (weight/height^2). These are simple and use little in the way of equipment (scale, non-stretchable tape measure, calipers) but require close attention to calibration and standardization, including both replicate variability and interobserver differences. More direct measures of body composition involves the assessment of the various fluid compartments, lean body mass (or non-fat mass), and fat mass. The methods include body density determinations (underwater weighing) for fat mass, total body potassium (by exchangeable potassium or whole body radioactive counting for the natural isotope ^{40}K) to assess lean body mass, total body nitrogen, total body electrical conductivity, magnetic resonance or computerized axial tomography studies to measure fat and muscle mass, dual photon absorptiometry, and bioelectric impedance analysis (BIA). These measures are highly correlated with one another, and when studied, with actual tissue analysis on cadavers. With the exception of BIA, these studies are more technical, and in some instances use instrumentation available only in specialized research centers.

BIA is simple, portable, uses no radioactivity, is without risk and is field friendly. BIA uses a small hand-carried instrument to generate a current, delivered to the body via two upper limb electrodes, and measures resistance and capacitive resistance (usually termed reactance) at two lower limb electrodes. Resistance to the flow of current is determined by the salt and water containing fat-free compartments, whereas reactance is the storage of charge, presumed to be the cell membrane, the biological equivalent of an electrical capacitor with a polar protein core sandwiched between two non-polar lipid bilayers. The data are transformed into body composition by nomograms which vary according to sex, age, height and weight, but according to recent studies, not significantly with race. The correlation coefficient of BIA with standard assessments of body composition is > 0.9.

BIA has been employed in the course of studies in Africa intended to determine the cause of SLIM disease in Kinshasa, Zaire.[2] In one study, 200 consecutive adult patients admitted to the Mama Yemo Hospital were examined. The mean age of the males was 38 years, 59% were HIV positive, the mean CD4 count was 428 and 54% died within three weeks in the hospital. The mean age of the women was 34, 67% were HIV positive, the mean CD4 count was 376, and 35% died in a hospital. When stratified by HIV status, both groups had lost considerable weight, with a relative increase in total body water, and more severe wasting of lean body mass in the AIDS patients. Symptoms of dysphagia or evidence of severe oral candidiasis was associated with a relative increase in the depletion of fat mass, primarily in women, similar to findings in the U.S. using more sophisticated techniques. When CD4 count was stratified by wasting determined by BIA, whether HIV associated or not, the two groups overlapped. The conclusion was that severe malnutrition associated with end-stage chronic disease causes a loss of CD4 cells (and inversion of the CD4/CD8 ratio) similar to AIDS. Thus, the only sure way to distinguish between the HIV infected and non-infected but chronically ill subjects was by serological testing. The in-hospital mortality rate was around 40% in HIV negative subjects, rose to approximately 60% in the HIV infected, and was significantly higher when acid-fast bacilli were detected in the stool by Ziehl-Neelson stain or by auramine fluorescence.

Prospective and cross-sectional studies in Zaire have shown that changes in body composition begin early and are progressive. A study comparing healthy HIV negative women, asymptomatic women known to be HIV seropositive for at least 5 years, and a group of women with advanced HIV infection showed progressive weight loss, decrease in biceps, triceps and subscapular skinfold thickness, decrease in mid-arm circumference, alteration in BIA resistance indicative of loss of lean body mass, albumin and carotene. The absolute CD4 cell count and CD4/CD8 ratio in the three groups were 944 and 1.44, 482 and 0.44, and 360 and 0.38, respectively, demonstrating the progression of HIV infection in these women. A striking finding was the marked elevation of cytokines in plasma in the asymptomatically infected women, equivalent to those seen with endotoxin infusion or in burn patients. Most dramatic was the rise in two natural cytokine antagonists, s-TNFR, the soluble TNF-receptor, and IL-IRa, the IL-I receptor antagonist. Thus, the ratio of s-TNFR to TNF was 57.4 in the asymptomatically infected women compared to 1.8 in the AIDS patients. Similarly, the IL-IRa to IL-1 was 11.6 in the former and 1.8 in the latter group. Levels of interferon gamma correlated with fever, and were more often detected in the AIDS patients, indicating that they were not "burned-out" and incapable of responding. These data suggest that the early evidence of wasting is correlated with evidence of early activation of cytokines, presumably due to the replication of HIV known to be occurring in the lymph nodes in the "latent" phase of HIV infection, but that symptoms of cytokine production are controlled by antagonist proteins. It may be that the ratio of antagonist to agonist cytokine determines the extent of the metabolic changes that lead to loss of lean and fat mass. The effect of superimposed infection was not studied, however it is possible that such infections might preferentially increase the agonist cytokines, since infection increases the consumption of body protein and resting energy expenditure, which continues into the chronic phase, in contrast to simple starvation, which is characterized by both protein sparing and reduced resting energy expenditure.

Further studies of the mechanisms of wasting in this same African population have revealed a high frequency of *Helicobacter pylori* infection and achlorhydria, increasing host susceptibility to intestinal infection, evidence of small bowel overgrowth by duodenal intubation and culture and hydrogen breath tests in around 1/3 of patients with chronic diarrhea, with evidence of fat malabsorption in around 20%, and increases in intestinal mucosal permeability assessed by the mannitol/lactulose test. Routine bacterial pathogens, primarily *Shigella* and *Salmonella*, were found in 21%. Thus, of the potential mechanisms of wasting, studies in one developing country have documented the presence of anorexia, dysphagia, weakness and lethargy as causes of decreased nutrient intake, defects in intestinal permeability, specific infections and small bowel overgrowth as causes of malabsorption, and catabolic responses and evidence for cytokine mediated metabolic changes as causes of endogenous metabolic disturbances.

TUBERCULOSIS AND HIV IN THE DEVELOPING WORLD

Mycobacterium tuberculosis is probably the most common opportunistic infection in AIDS patients in the developing world. In recent studies, 2/3 of the patients with tuberculosis in Kampala, Uganda were HIV positive, and these individuals had more prominent histories of fever and weight loss. A 32-month follow-up of HIV positive Ziarean women revealed a risk of tuberculosis of 3.1 per 100 person-years in the HIV infected compared to 0.12 per 100 person-years in the HIV uninfected, a relative risk of 26 attributable to HIV infection. A number of studies have documented an annual risk of active tuberculosis of 5-8% in HIV infected individuals in developing countries. Modeling studies suggest that, depending on the prevalence of latent tuberculous infection in the general population, ranging from 45-60%, and the prevalence of HIV, ranging from 2-20%, somewhere between a 40% and a 620% increase in the tuberculosis incidence rates will happen between 1980, pre-HIV, and 2000, well into the epidemic. It is not only of interest, but of likely importance, that both HIV and tuberculosis cause wasting, SLIM disease and consumption, and that both cause energy and a reduction of the PPD skin test response, associated with a loss of cell-mediated immune responses.

Thus, malnutrition develops early in HIV positive patients in developing countries, with a pattern of body composition changes similar to U.S. and European patients. Also, severe malnutrition in HIV negative patients results in depressed CD4 cell number which overlaps that found in HIV positive patients with wasting syndrome. Mortality rates are high in both groups. Early exuberant cytokine responses may be checked by concomitant anti-inflammatory cytokine responses. The balance of the two may determine the cytokine-mediated metabolic changes resulting in catabolism and altered anabolism. Indeed, most potential mechanisms for wasting syndrome have been documented in AIDS patients in developing countries. Further, the benefits of nutritional therapy in the developing country setting has yet to be demonstrated, but if effective in blunting the wasting response, nutritional therapy could have an effect on the incidence of active tuberculosis.

REFERENCES

1. Keusch, G.T. and Thea, D.M. (1993). Malnutrition and AIDS. Med. Clin. North Am. 77(4): 795-814.

2. Hassig, S.E., Perriens, J., Baende, E., and Kahotwa, M. (1990). An analysis of the economic impact of HIV infection among patients at Mama Yemo Hospital, Kinshasa, Zaire. AIDS 4:883-887.

Tuberculosis
and the Nutritionally Disadvantaged: Conclusions

Frank M. Collins, PhD, DSc

M. tuberculosis is a highly infectious human pathogen which is spread person-to-person by means of droplet infection from a patient with open cavitary disease. Tuberculin conversion rates in a closed environment (nursing home, prison, homeless shelter) can be extraordinarily high unless the index case is identified and treated until no longer infectious. Most adults (90-95%) are innately resistant to tuberculosis, developing a latent form of the disease in which small numbers of virulent tubercle bacilli can persist within the tissues for long periods of time. This quiescent infection may later reactivate during old age or in individuals suffering from severe malnutrition, chronic alcoholism, drug abuse or HIV infection which ablate the normally effective cellular defenses. The mechanisms responsible for this loss of immunity are under active investigation using the sort of experimental approaches discussed by Drs. McMurray, Ross, and Chan during this roundtable. In addition to the direct effects that severe protein and Vitamin A deficiency have on

Frank M. Collins, Mycobacteria Laboratory, FDA, CBER, Bethesda, MD.
Address correspondence to: Frank M. Collins, PhD, DSc, Mycobacteria Laboratory, FDA, Center for Biological Evaluation and Research, Building 29, Room 129, 8800 Rockville Pike, Bethesda, MD 20892.

[Haworth co-indexing entry note]: "Tuberculosis and the Nutritionally Disadvantaged: Conclusions." Collins, Frank M. Co-published simultaneously in *Journal of Nutritional Immunology* (The Haworth Medical Press, an imprint of The Haworth Press, Inc.) Vol. 5, No. 1, 1997, pp. 51-54; and: *Nutritional Abnormalities in Infectious Diseases: Effects on Tuberculosis and AIDS* (ed: Christopher E. Taylor) The Haworth Medical Press, an imprint of The Haworth Press, Inc., 1997, pp. 51-54. Single or multiple copies of this article are available for a fee from The Haworth Document Delivery Service [1-800-342-9678, 9:00 a.m. - 5:00 p.m. (EST). E-mail address: getinfo@haworth.com].

T-cell numbers and repertoire, prolonged malabsorption of nutrients (and drugs) as a result of heavy intestinal mucosal involvement by one of the more pathogenic members of the *M. avium*-complex can further complicate the picture. Histopathological examination of biopsy material taken from many AIDS patients reveals lesions not unlike that seen in Johne's disease in cattle or Whipple's disease in people. Prolonged malnutrition also adversely affects macrophage activity, a phenomenon seen in low birth-weight babies and HIV-infected patients with the "wasting' syndrome, contributing to the immunodeficiency discussed by Drs. Chan and Douglas in a laboratory setting and by Drs. Huitt and Cunningham-Rundles from a clinical viewpoint. Finally, Dr. Keusch discussed the double role played by malnutrition and HIV infection in many parts of Eastern Europe, Africa, India, and China, areas where tuberculosis is already well entrenched.[1]

From a more personal viewpoint, 1 find nothing new in the relationship between nutrition and tuberculosis: my mother knew all about it when she urged me to eat my carrots and greens so I wouldn't catch consumption. Years later, 1 listened to some of the old "lungers" still living in Saranac Lake reminisce about life at the Sanatorium in the "good old days," and was struck by their repeated reference to the rich food provided to the patients, with up to 6 meals a day, with all the meat, dairy products and eggs they could handle (blood cholesterol levels were the least of their worries in those days). In addition, they were encouraged to sunbathe (or to sit in front of an ultraviolet lamp) which we now know increases the production of Vitamin D leading to enhanced macrophage tuberculocidal activity.[2] So, it is nice to have a scientific rationale for these earlier empirical observations.

It is ironic that we may be forced to return to some of these non-specific therapeutic measures in order to "cure" patients infected with multidrug-resistant tubercle bacilli which they acquired as nosocomial infection in the AIDS or tuberculosis ward. Some of these strains are resistant to 6 or more drugs, with good epidemiological and experimental data to indicate that they retain both infectiousness and virulence. The pathogenicity of these organisms for AIDS patients can be awesome, with death occurring before the drug resistance pattern is established by a diagnostic laboratory.

However, AIDS patients are not the only ones being infected by these MDR-TB. There are a number of reports of tuberculous infections in health care workers (HCW), social workers, prison guards, and homeless shelter personnel.[3] The tubercle bacillus has always been a notorious laboratory pathogen, so it is hardly surprising that tuberculin conversions are occurring in HCWs and laboratory personnel exposed to these MDR-TB. How many of these individuals will eventually develop drug-resistant disease is uncertain, but several deaths have already been reported.

The number of multidrug-resistant isolates of *M. tuberculosis* reported to the CDC has risen sharply from around 1% in 1981 to nearly 7% by 1991, with isolation rates in some inner city hospitals running as high as 30%. Several outbreaks of MDR-TB in prison systems from around the country are raising questions as to the best way to prevent such outbreaks in the future. Tuberculosis control in this country has traditionally relied on case finding and drug treatment and the standard protocol of isoniazid, rifampin, ethambutol and pyrazinamide achieves sputum negativity within a matter of weeks, although treatment must be continued for another 6 months in order to prevent relapses. Contacts are screened by tuberculin skin testing and any converters are placed on isoniazid therapy for 6 months. This strategy has been highly effective in communities with a low annual exposure rate and predominantly drug-sensitive organisms. However, when HIV and MDR-TB are added to the equation, more complex, expensive and toxic drug regimens must be used, with an increased risk of non-compliance and further drug resistance. Given the increasing number of AIDS patients reported in the United States each year and their predilection for mycobacterial involvement, it seems likely that both diseases will continue to be important public health problems in this country for many years to come.

The presence of MDR-TB in the community calls for the development of new, more effective diagnostic, prophylactic and therapeutic reagents. However, innovative approaches to this problem have been limited by a paucity of epidemiological and immunological data on the *in vivo* behavior of these drug-resistant pathogens. We need to learn a lot more about the host-parasite interactions responsible for the development of latent tuberculosis. Also, what is the most effective way to prevent the spread of MDR-TB infections in the county jails, in hospital wards, in the home? Should BCG vaccination be required for all tuberculin negative personnel working in tuberculosis and AIDS wards? What are the relative merits of BCG vaccination vs. regular skin testing in the face of increasing drug resistance? Is the loss of tuberculin sensitivity by BCG-vaccinated individuals worth acquiring an uncertain level of resistance to MDR-TB infection. A recent meta-analysis of BCG field trial data indicates an average of 50% protection in vaccinated children and adults.[4] Even a 50% reduction in active disease in staff working with AIDS patients infected with MDR-TB would seem desirable.[5] Should BCG vaccination be offered to people (especially infants) living under conditions of high exposure, poor nutrition, and minimal health care? What options should be offered to tuberculin negative, HIV-infected individuals who are at risk of developing MDR-TB or *M. avium*-complex disease? What is the significance of a "doubtful" skin reaction to PPD (5-9 mm induration) in such individuals? HIV-infected individuals cannot be vaccinated with live BCG and as such inactivated preparation with immunotherapeutic properties will be needed if we are to bring this epidemic under control in the foreseeable future.[6]

REFERENCES

1. Stanford, J.L., Grange, J.M., and Pozniak, A. (1991). Is Africa lost? Lancet. 338:557-558.

2. Rook, G.A. W., Steele, I., and Fraher, L. (1986). Vitamin D3, gamma interferon and control of proliferation of *Mycobacterium tuberculosis* by human monocytes. Immunol. 57:159-163.

3. Centers for Disease Control. (1991). Nosocomial transmission of multidrug-resistant tuberculosis among HIV-infected persons–Florida and New York 1981-1991. MMWR 40:585-591.

4. Colditz, G.A., Brewer, T.F., and Berkey, C.S. (1994). Efficacy of BCG vaccine in the prevention of tuberculosis. JAMA 271:698-702.

5. Greenberg, P.D., Lax, K.G., and Schechter, C.B. (1991). Tuberculosis in house staff. A decision analysis comparing the tuberculin screening strategy with the BCG vaccination. Amer. Rev. Resp. Dis. 143: 490-495.

6. Stanford, J.L. and Grange, J.M. (1993). New concepts for the control of tuberculosis in the twenty-first century. J. Roy. Coll. Physicians, Lond. 27: 218-223.

Index

Page numbers followed by "t" denote tables and "f" denote figures.

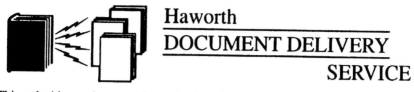

Haworth
DOCUMENT DELIVERY
SERVICE

This valuable service provides a single-article order form for any article from a Haworth journal.

- *Time Saving:* No running around from library to library to find a specific article.
- *Cost Effective:* All costs are kept down to a minimum.
- *Fast Delivery:* Choose from several options, including same-day FAX.
- *No Copyright Hassles:* You will be supplied by the original publisher.
- *Easy Payment:* Choose from several easy payment methods.

Open Accounts Welcome for . . .
- Library Interlibrary Loan Departments
- Library Network/Consortia Wishing to Provide Single-Article Services
- Indexing/Abstracting Services with Single Article Provision Services
- Document Provision Brokers and Freelance Information Service Providers

---

MAIL or *FAX* THIS ENTIRE ORDER FORM TO:

Haworth Document Delivery Service
The Haworth Press, Inc.
10 Alice Street
Binghamton, NY 13904-1580

or FAX: 1-800-895-0582
or CALL: 1-800-342-9678
9am-5pm EST

PLEASE SEND ME PHOTOCOPIES OF THE FOLLOWING SINGLE ARTICLES:

1) Journal Title: _____

   Vol/Issue/Year:_____Starting & Ending Pages:_____

   Article Title:_____

2) Journal Title: _____

   Vol/Issue/Year:_____Starting & Ending Pages:_____

   Article Title:_____

3) Journal Title: _____

   Vol/Issue/Year:_____Starting & Ending Pages:_____

   Article Title:_____

4) Journal Title: _____

   Vol/Issue/Year:_____Starting & Ending Pages:_____

   Article Title:_____

(See other side for Costs and Payment Information)

COSTS: Please figure your cost to order quality copies of an article.

1. Set-up charge per article: $8.00
   ($8.00 × number of separate articles)   _____

2. Photocopying charge for each article:

   1-10 pages: $1.00   _____

   11-19 pages: $3.00   _____

   20-29 pages: $5.00   _____

   30+ pages: $2.00/10 pages   _____

3. Flexicover (optional): $2.00/article   _____

4. Postage & Handling: US: $1.00 for the first article/
   $.50 each additional article   _____

   Federal Express: $25.00   _____

   Outside US: $2.00 for first article/
   $.50 each additional article _____

5. Same-day FAX service: $.35 per page   _____

   GRAND TOTAL: _____

METHOD OF PAYMENT: (please check one)

❑ Check enclosed   ❑ Please ship and bill. PO # _____
(sorry we can ship and bill to bookstores only! All others must pre-pay)

❑ Charge to my credit card: ❑ Visa; ❑ MasterCard; ❑ Discover;
❑ American Express;

Account Number:_____ Expiration date:_____

Signature: X_____

Name: _____ Institution: _____

Address: _____

_____

City: _____ State:_____ Zip:_____

Phone Number: _____ FAX Number: _____

MAIL or *FAX* THIS ENTIRE ORDER FORM TO:

Haworth Document Delivery Service	**or FAX: 1-800-895-0582**
The Haworth Press, Inc.	**or CALL: 1-800-342-9678**
10 Alice Street	9am-5pm EST)
Binghamton, NY 13904-1580	